OB/GYN Emergencies

Editors

SARAH K. SOMMERKAMP
KATHLEEN WITTELS

EMERGENCY MEDICINE CLINICS OF NORTH AMERICA

www.emed.theclinics.com

Consulting Editor
AMAL MATTU

November 2012 • Volume 30 • Number 4

ELSEVIER

1600 John F. Kennedy Boulevard ● Suite 1800 ● Philadelphia, Pennsylvania 19103-2899

http://www.theclinics.com

EMERGENCY MEDICINE CLINICS OF NORTH AMERICA Volume 30, Number 4
November 2012 ISSN 0733-8627, ISBN-13: 978-1-4557-5835-7

Editor: Patrick Manley
Developmental Editor: Donald Mumford

Emergency Medicine Clinics of North America (ISSN 0733-8627) is published quarterly by Elsevier Inc., 360 Park Avenue South, New York, NY, 10010-1710. Months of issue are February, May, August, and November. Business and Editorial Offices: 1600 John F. Kennedy Boulevard, Suite 1800, Philadelphia, PA 19103-2899. Customer Service Office: 6277 Sea Harbor Drive, Orlando, FL 32887-4800. Periodicals postage paid at New York, NY, and additional mailing offices. Subscription prices are $142.00 per year (US students), $281.00 per year (US individuals), $478.00 per year (US institutions), $201.00 per year (international students), $404.00 per year (international individuals), $576.00 per year (international institutions), $201.00 per year (Canadian students), $347.00 per year (Canadian individuals), and $576.00 per year (Canadian institutions). International air speed delivery is included in all *Clinics'* subscription prices. All prices are subject to change without notice. **POSTMASTER:** Send address changes to *Emergency Medicine Clinics of North America*, Elsevier Periodicals Customer Service, 11830 Westline Industrial Drive, St. Louis, MO 63146. Customer Service (orders, claims, online, change of address): Elsevier Periodicals Customer Service, 11830 Westline Industrial Drive, St. Louis, MO 63146. Tel: 1-800-654-2452 (U.S. and Canada); 314-453-7041 (outside U.S. and Canada). Fax: 314-453-5170. E-mail: journalscustomerservice-usa@elsevier.com (for print support); journalsonline support-usa@elsevier.com (for online support).

Reprints. For copies of 100 or more of articles in this publication, please contact the Commercial Reprints Department, Elsevier Inc., 360 Park Avenue South, New York, NY 10010-1710. Tel.: 212-633-3812; Fax: 212-462-1935; E-mail: reprints@elsevier.com.

Emergency Medicine Clinics of North America is covered in *MEDLINE/PubMed (Index Medicus), Current Contents/Clinical Medicine, EMBASE/Excerpta Medica, BIOSIS, SciSearch, CINAHL, ISI/BIOMED,* and *Research Alert.*

Printed and bound by CPI Group (UK) Ltd, Croydon, CR0 4YY

Transferred to digital print 2012

Contributors

CONSULTING EDITOR

AMAL MATTU, MD
Professor and Vice Chair, Department of Emergency Medicine, University of Maryland School of Medicine, Baltimore, Maryland

GUEST EDITORS

SARAH K. SOMMERKAMP, MD, RDMS
Assistant professor, Department of Emergency Medicine, University of Maryland School of Medicine; Director of Emergency Ultrasound, Maryland General Hospital, Baltimore, Maryland

KATHLEEN WITTELS, MD
Assistant Medical Director, STRATUS Center for Medical Simulation, Department of Emergency Medicine, Brigham and Women's Hospital, Boston, Massachusetts

AUTHORS

STEPHEN J. CIPOT, DO
Resident in Emergency Medicine, Department of Emergency Medicine, Northshore University Hospital, Manhasset, New York

ANGELA R. CIRILLI, MD, RDMS
Department of Emergency Medicine, North Shore University Hospital, Manhasset, New York; Assistant Professor of Emergency Medicine, Hofstra Northshore–LIJ School of Medicine, Hempstead, New York

TERESA M. DEAK, MD
Resident, Department of Emergency Medicine, North Shore University Hospital, Manhasset, New York

LAURA DIEGELMANN, MD, RDMS
Clinical Instructor, Department of Emergency Medicine, University of Maryland School of Medicine, Baltimore, Maryland

BRIAN D. EUERLE, MD, RDMS
Associate Professor, Department of Emergency Medicine, University of Maryland School of Medicine, Baltimore, Maryland

ALISA GIBSON, MD, DMD
Clinical Assistant Professor, Department of Emergency Medicine, University of Maryland School of Medicine, Baltimore, Maryland

SAM HSU, MD, RDMS
Assistant Professor, Department of Emergency Medicine, University of Maryland School of Medicine, Baltimore, Maryland

NADIA HUANCAHUARI, MD
Clinical Instructor, Harvard Medical School; Department of Emergency Medicine, Brigham and Women's Hospital, Boston, Massachusetts

MEGAN C. KING, DO
Chief Resident, Family Medicine Department, Medstar Franklin Square Medical Center, Baltimore, Maryland

MICHAEL LEVINE, MD
Assistant Professor, Section of Medical Toxicology, Department of Emergency Medicine, University of Southern California, Los Angeles, California; Attending Physician, Department of Medical Toxicology, Banner Good Samaritan Medical Center, Phoenix, Arizona

DAVID MEGUERDICHIAN, MD
Clinical Instructor in Medicine (Emergency Medicine), Harvard Medical School; Attending Physician, Department of Emergency Medicine, Brigham and Women's Hospital, Boston, Massachusetts

SIAMAK MOAYEDI, MD
Assistant Professor, Department of Emergency Medicine, University of Maryland School of Medicine, Baltimore, Maryland

JOSHUA B. MOSKOVITZ, MD, MPH
Department of Emergency Medicine, North Shore University Hospital, Manhasset, New York; Assistant Professor of Emergency Medicine, Department of Emergency Medicine, Hofstra North Shore-LIJ School of Medicine, Hempstead, New York

AYRN D. O'CONNOR, MD
Assistant Professor, Department of Emergency Medicine, University of Arizona School of Medicine, Phoenix, Arizona; Department of Medical Toxicology, Banner Good Samaritan Medical Center, Phoenix, Arizona

KAREN E. PERKINS, MD
Director, Maternal Child Health Curriculum, Family Medicine Department, Medstar Franklin Square Medical Center, Baltimore, Maryland; Presently, Faculty, Family Medicine Residency, Carilion Clinic, Roanoke, Virginia

ALI S. RAJA, MD, MBA, MPH
Associate Director for Trauma, Department of Emergency Medicine, Brigham and Women's Hospital, Harvard Medical School, Boston, Massachusetts

FRANK SABATINO, MD
Assistant Professor of Emergency Medicine, Hofstra North Shore–LIJ School of Medicine, Hempstead, New York; Department of Emergency Medicine, North Shore University Hospital, Manhasset, New York

DAVID W. SILVER, MD, MA
Assistant Professor of Emergency Medicine, Hofstra North Shore–LIJ School of Medicine, Hempstead, New York; Department of Emergency Medicine, North Shore University Hospital, Manhasset, New York

SARAH K. SOMMERKAMP, MD, RDMS
Assistant Professor, Department of Emergency Medicine, University of Maryland School of Medicine, Baltimore, Maryland

MERCEDES TORRES, MD
Clinical Assistant Professor, Department of Emergency Medicine, University of Maryland School of Medicine, Baltimore, Maryland

CHRISTOPHER P. ZABBO, DO
Program Director, Emergency Medicine Residency, Kent Hospital/UNECOM; EM Ultrasound Director, Department of Emergency Medicine, Kent Hospital, Warwick, Rhode Island; Clinical Assistant Professor, Department of Emergency Medicine, UNECOM, Biddeford, Maine

Contents

First-trimester vaginal bleeding and abdominal pain are common complaints in the emergency department. The differential diagnosis is broad, ranging from benign conditions to life-threatening complications. This is a difficult topic because it is charged not only with immediate emotional connotations but also with potential long-term effects on the patient's ability to become pregnant again. This article reviews the presentation, diagnosis, and management of implantation bleeding, subchorionic hemorrhage, spontaneous abortion, ectopic pregnancy, heterotopic pregnancy, anembryonic pregnancy, hyperemesis gravidarum, gestational trophoblastic disease, and round ligament syndrome.

For the emergency physician tasked with evaluating the patient with an obstetric emergency, ultrasound can provide important and potentially lifesaving information. Ultrasound of the pregnant patient is unique in that two possible approaches can be used: transabdominal and transvaginal. Another unique feature is that an understanding of developmental anatomy, which changes during pregnancy, is important. Two of the most basic yet important uses of ultrasound in the pregnant patient are to provide information concerning the gestational age of the pregnancy and the fetal heart rate. Ultrasound has a major role in the diagnosis and management of the patient with a suspected ectopic pregnancy.

The treatment of gynecologic and other infections in obstetric patients involves consideration of the physiologic changes of pregnancy, the clinical implications of the infection for the patient as well as the fetus, and the safety of antimicrobials available for therapy. This article highlights the treatment of infections of the vagina, uterus, and urinary tract, with a focus on how therapy changes in obstetric patients. In addition, the emergency department management of other clinically important infections in pregnancy, such as those caused by the human immunodeficiency virus, influenza viruses, methicillin-resistant *Staphylococcus aureus, Parvovirus, Listeria*, and others is reviewed.

The focus of this article is the evaluation and management of pregnant patients with nonobstetric abdominal pain and surgical emergencies. The anatomic and physiologic changes that occur during pregnancy can cause difficulties in interpreting patients' signs and symptoms in emergency departments. This article reviews some of the common causes of nonobstetric abdominal pain and surgical emergencies that present to emergency departments and discusses some of the literature surrounding the use of imaging modalities during pregnancy. After a review of these changes and their causes, imaging modalities that can be used for the assessment are discussed.

Hypertension in pregnancy is increasing in prevalence and incidence and its treatment becoming more commonplace. Associated complications of pregnancy, including end-organ damage, preeclampsia, eclampsia, and postpartum eclampsia, are leading sources of maternal and fetal morbidity and mortality, requiring an emergency physician to become proficient with their identification and treatment. This article reviews hypertension in pregnancy as it relates to outcomes, with special emphasis on preeclampsia, eclampsia, and postpartum eclampsia.

Complications of late pregnancy are managed infrequently in the emergency department and, thus, can pose a challenge when the emergency physician encounters acute presentations. An expert understanding of the anatomic and physiologic changes and possible complications of late pregnancy is vital to ensure proper evaluation and care for both mother and fetus. This article focuses on the late pregnancy issues that the emergency physician will face, from the bleeding and instability of abruptio placentae to the wide spectrum of complications and management strategies encountered with preterm labor.

The treatment of pregnant patients with traumatic injuries requires knowledge of the fundamentals of general trauma management as well as the specific anatomic and physiologic changes brought about by pregnancy. This article provides a review of the spectrum of trauma prevention and treatment in pregnant women, from counseling strategies that can be used during any emergency department visit to a step-by-step evaluation protocol for patients with trauma during pregnancy and the severe injuries that might be encountered by providers during the treatment of these women, including maternal cardiopulmonary arrest and the perimortem cesarean section.

Cardiovascular emergencies in pregnancy are rare but often catastrophic. This article reviews the diagnosis and management of venous thromboembolism, aortic dissection, acquired heart disease and cardiomyopathy, acute myocardial infarction, and cardiac dysrhythmias in the setting of pregnancy. It also reviews updated resuscitation guidelines for cardiac arrest and perimortem cesarean section.

Any delivery in the emergency department is considered a precipitous birth and is an anxiety-producing event. Many deliveries proceed without incident. However, the emergency physician must be prepared for several dreaded scenarios, such as nuchal cord, shoulder dystocia, and breech birth. This article reviews the basics, complications, and management of such deliveries.

The emergency physician frequently encounters women who seek care because of pregnancy- and nonpregnancy-related complaints. Many medications are safe for use during pregnancy, including several that are listed as potential teratogens based on the Food and Drug Administration's (FDA) pregnancy classification; but it is important that the emergency physician know and recognize which drugs can be given in pregnancy and which drugs are absolutely contraindicated. Expert resources should be identified and used because the FDA's classification of drugs based on pregnancy risk does not represent the most up-to-date or accurate assessment of a drug's safety.

Evaluation of the nonpregnant patient presenting to the emergency department with vaginal bleeding requires the emergency physician to be aware of the potential for a variety of underlying causes. Patients with vaginal bleeding may have non–life-threatening problems such as fibroids, endometriosis, or treatable sexually transmitted diseases such as gonorrhea and chlamydial infection. However, care must be taken to differentiate these from more serious causes of pelvic pain and bleeding such as ectopic pregnancy, hemorrhagic cyst, ovarian torsion, and rare complications from fibroids such as intraperitoneal hemorrhage. Abnormal bleeding unrelated to structural problems could have an anovulatory or ovulatory cause.

Most postmenopausal vaginal bleeding is benign; however, it merits diagnostic evaluation by transvaginal ultrasound or endometrial biopsy after emergency department evaluation. Patients and physicians may treat menopausal symptoms with hormone replacement therapy or other agents, such as venlafaxine or gabapentin. Hormone replacement therapy, when initiated close to the start of menopause and continued at the lowest possible dose for the shortest possible duration, carries less risk than previously believed. Pelvic organ prolapse affects millions of women and may contribute to poor body image and difficulty with urinary, gastrointestinal, and sexual function. Treatment options include Kegel exercises, pessaries, and surgery.

EMERGENCY MEDICINE CLINICS OF NORTH AMERICA

GOAL STATEMENT
The goal of *Emergency Medicine Clinics of North America* is to keep practicing physicians up to date with current clinical practice in emergency medicine by providing timely articles reviewing the state of the art in patient care.

ACCREDITATION
The *Emergency Medical Clinics of North America* is planned and implemented in accordance with the Essential Areas and Policies of the Accreditation Council for Continuing Medical Education (ACCME) through the joint sponsorship of the University of Virginia School of Medicine and Elsevier. The University of Virginia School of Medicine is accredited by the ACCME to provide continuing medical education for physicians.

The University of Virginia School of Medicine designates this enduring material activity for a maximum of 15 *AMA PRA Category 1 Credit*(s)™ for each issue, 60 credits per year. Physicians should claim only the credit commensurate with the extent of their participation in the activity.

The American Medical Association has determined that physicians not licensed in the US who participate in this CME enduring material activity are eligible for a maximum of 15 *AMA PRA Category 1 Credit*(s)™ for each issue, 60 credits per year.

The Emergency Medicine Clinics of North America CME program is approved by the American College of Emergency Physicians for 60 hours of ACEP Category I Credit per year.

Credit can be earned by reading the text material, taking the CME examination online at http://www.theclinics.com/home/cme, and completing the evaluation. After taking the test, you will be required to review any and all incorrect answers. Following completion of the test and evaluation, your credit will be awarded and you may print your certificate.

FACULTY DISCLOSURE/CONFLICT OF INTEREST
The University of Virginia School of Medicine, as an ACCME accredited provider, endorses and strives to comply with the Accreditation Council for Continuing Medical Education (ACCME) Standards of Commercial Support, Commonwealth of Virginia statutes, University of Virginia policies and procedures, and associated federal and private regulations and guidelines on the need for disclosure and monitoring of proprietary and financial interests that may affect the scientific integrity and balance of content delivered in continuing medical education activities under our auspices.

The University of Virginia School of Medicine requires that all CME activities accredited through this institution be developed independently and be scientifically rigorous, balanced and objective in the presentation/discussion of its content, theories and practices.

All authors/editors participating in an accredited CME activity are expected to disclose to the readers relevant financial relationships with commercial entities occurring within the past 12 months (such as grants or research support, employee, consultant, stock holder, member of speakers bureau, etc.). The University of Virginia School of Medicine will employ appropriate mechanisms to resolve potential conflicts of interest to maintain the standards of fair and balanced education to the reader. Questions about specific strategies can be directed to the Office of Continuing Medical Education, University of Virginia School of Medicine, Charlottesville, Virginia.

The faculty and staff of the University of Virginia Office of Continuing Medical Education have no financial affiliations to disclose.

The authors/editors listed below have identified no professional or financial affiliations for themselves or their spouse/partner:
Stephen J. Cipot, DO; Angela R. Cirilli, MD, RDMS; Teresa M. Deak, MD; Laura Diegelmann, MD, RDMS; Brian D. Euerle, MD, RDMS; Alisa Gibson, MD, DMD; Sam Hsu, MD, RDMS; Nadia Huancahuari, MD; Megan C. King, DO; Michael Levine, MD; Patrick Manley, (Acquisitions Editor); Amal Mattu, MD (Consulting Editor); David Meguerdichian, MD; Siamak Moayedi, MD; Joshua B. Moskovitz, MD, MPH; Ayrn D. O'Connor, MD; Karen E. Perkins, MD; Frank Sabatino, MD; David W. Silver, MD, MA; Sarah K. Sommerkamp, MD, RDMS (Guest Editor); Mercedes Torres, MD; Kathleen Wittels, MD (Guest Editor); William A. Woods, MD (Test Author); and Christopher P. Zabbo, DO.

The authors/editors listed below identified the following professional or financial affiliations for themselves or their spouse/partner:
Ali S. Raja, MD, MBA, MPH is on the Advisory Board for Diagnotion, LLC.

Disclosure of Discussion of Non-FDA Approved Uses for Pharmaceutical Products and/or Medical Devices.
The University of Virginia School of Medicine, as an ACCME provider, requires that all faculty presenters identify and disclose any off-label uses for pharmaceutical and medical device products. The University of Virginia School of Medicine recommends that each physician fully review all the available data on new products or procedures prior to clinical use.

TO ENROLL
To enroll in the Emergency Medicine Clinics of North America Continuing Medical Education program, call customer service at 1-800-654-2452 or visit us online at www.theclinics.com/home/cme. The CME program is available to subscribers for an additional fee of $190.00.

Foreword

Obstetric and Gynecological Emergencies

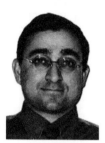

Amal Mattu, MD
Consulting Editor

A typical shift in a busy emergency department (ED) would easily involve the management of conditions such as myocardial infarction, congestive heart failure, stroke, abdominal surgical conditions, multisystem trauma, fractures, gunshot wounds, and shock. Trained emergency physicians rarely bat an eye when these conditions present. In fact, we *live* for these high-intensity scenarios.

Everything changes, however, with the arrival of a pregnant woman in active labor. Calm becomes chaos in the ED, and the thrill of intensity quickly becomes dysphoria. I encountered such a scenario during my last shift, and amid the anxiety I felt, I realized the irony: I would rather have been managing a patient with almost any other medical illness than this patient who was involved in a totally natural act that had played out countless times since the evolution of humans. Mom pushed; the baby cried, and we all felt relieved to be able to go back to seeing the *sick* patients. Needless to say, when pregnant patients present to the ED, they often engender a significant sense of uneasiness among the providers, despite their usual baseline health.

In this issue of *Emergency Medicine Clinics of North America*, guest editors Drs Sarah Sommerkamp and Kathleen Wittels have assembled an outstanding group of authors to educate us on this vital aspect of our specialty. Articles discuss emergencies in early, mid, and late pregnancy. Infections, teratogens, trauma, cardiovascular disorders, and nonobstetric surgical emergencies are discussed in detail relevant to emergency medicine. An article is devoted to precipitous and difficult deliveries, and a separate article is devoted to ultrasound imaging in pregnancy. Two separate articles are also provided to address high-risk conditions in the nonpregnant female patient: vaginal bleeding and geriatric gynecology.

This issue of *Emergency Medicine Clinics of North America* represents an important addition to the emergency medicine literature. Drs Sommerkamp, Wittels, and their colleagues have provided a cutting-edge update on emergency obstetric care with additional selected gynecologic conditions. Emergency physicians in every type of

Emerg Med Clin N Am 30 (2012) xiii–xiv
http://dx.doi.org/10.1016/j.emc.2012.10.002
0733-8627/12/$ – see front matter

practice setting will find this issue immensely useful for those anxiety-provoking conditions when the pregnant patient arrives in the ED. Kudos to the contributors for an outstanding issue!

Amal Mattu, MD
Department of Emergency Medicine
University of Maryland School of Medicine
110 South Paca Street, Sixth Floor
Suite 200, Baltimore, MD 21201, USA

E-mail address:
amattu@smail.umaryland.edu

Preface

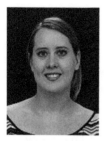 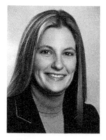

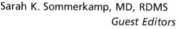

Sarah K. Sommerkamp, MD, RDMS   Kathleen Wittels, MD
Guest Editors

We are grateful for the opportunity to guest edit this edition of *Emergency Medicine Clinics of North America* on obstetric and gynecologic emergencies. This issue is written for emergency physicians in both academic and community practice. Recognizing that the range of support for obstetric conditions varies substantially at different facilities, our goal was to encompass both the common and the potentially catastrophic issues facing the emergency physician. Patients with obstetric emergencies can be some of the most stressful that the emergency physician encounters. The situations are frequently emotionally charged and the physician needs to consider the treatment effects on 2 patients. This issue covers problems faced in all trimesters of pregnancy as well as trauma, infections, and non-pregnancy-related abdominal pain in the pregnant woman. It also describes special considerations regarding medications and teratogens. The gynecologic problems covered are topics that focus on bleeding complaints and the less frequently discussed topic of geriatric gynecology. Our goal is to ensure the emergency physician is prepared with current literature and best practices. The topics in obstetrics and gynecology covered in this *Emergency Medicine Clinics of North America* range from urgent care complaints that are encountered daily to the highly stressful and potentially life-threatening events that are less frequently encountered but require the emergency physician to be ready to act. We hope that you enjoy!

We would like to express our gratitude to Amal Mattu, MD, and Patrick Manley for the opportunity to work on this project. We would like to express sincere thanks to all of the

Emerg Med Clin N Am 30 (2012) xv–xvi
http://dx.doi.org/10.1016/j.emc.2012.10.001
0733-8627/12/$ – see front matter © 2012 Elsevier Inc. All rights reserved.

emed.theclinics.com

authors for their hard work and diligence. We would also like to thank Christopher A. Floccare, editorial intern, and Linda J. Kesselring, MS, ELS, technical editor/writer, for their editorial support.

Sarah K. Sommerkamp, MD, RDMS
Department of Emergency Medicine
University of Maryland School of Medicine
110 South Paca Street, Sixth Floor
Suite 200, Baltimore, MD 21201, USA

Kathleen Wittels, MD
STRATUS Center for Medical Simulation
Department of Emergency Medicine
Brigham and Women's Hospital
75 Francis Street, Neville House
Boston, MA 02115, USA

E-mail addresses:
ssommerkamp@gmail.com (S.K. Sommerkamp)
kwittels@partners.org (K. Wittels)

Emergencies in Early Pregnancy

Nadia Huancahuari, MD[a,b,*]

KEYWORDS

- Implantation bleeding • Subchorionic hemorrhage • Spontaneous abortion
- Ectopic pregnancy • Heterotopic pregnancy • Anembryonic pregnancy
- Hyperemesis gravidarum • Round ligament syndrome

KEY POINTS

- A pregnancy test should be obtained on any woman of childbearing age with abdominal pain or vaginal bleeding.
- A ruptured ectopic pregnancy with hemoperitoneum constitutes an obstetric emergency, and its management includes prompt resuscitation and operative intervention.
- The incidence of heterotopic pregnancies has increased significantly since the advent of assisted conception and in vitro fertilization.
- Hydatidiform molar pregnancies may lead to malignant disease such as choriocarcinoma.

INTRODUCTION

During early pregnancy, approximately one-fourth of women experience vaginal spotting or bleeding.[1] Emergency physicians must be adept at evaluating and managing the array of causes of those symptoms. Although some of the complications of these complaints are life-threatening, it is critical that emergency care providers recognize the immediate emotional nature of these presentations and the potential effects on the patient's future fertility. This article discusses the presentation, diagnosis, and management of implantation bleeding, subchorionic hemorrhage (SH), spontaneous abortion, ectopic pregnancy, heterotopic pregnancy (HP), anembryonic pregnancy, hyperemesis gravidarum (HG), gestational trophoblastic disease (GTD), and round ligament syndrome.

There is no funding support for this article. The author has nothing to disclose.
[a] Harvard Medical School, Boston, MA, USA; [b] Department of Emergency Medicine, Brigham and Women's Hospital, 75 Francis Street, Neville House, Boston, MA 02115, USA
* Corresponding author. Department of Emergency Medicine, Brigham and Women's Hospital, 75 Francis Street, Neville House, Boston, MA 02115.
E-mail address: nhuancahuari@partners.org

Emerg Med Clin N Am 30 (2012) 837–847
http://dx.doi.org/10.1016/j.emc.2012.08.005
0733-8627/12/$ – see front matter © 2012 Elsevier Inc. All rights reserved.

emed.theclinics.com

FIRST-TRIMESTER ABDOMINAL PAIN AND BLEEDING
Implantation Bleeding

Definition
Implantation bleeding occurs when the blastocyst, the fertilized ovum, attaches to the uterine lining. On average, it occurs 9 days (range, 6–12 days) after ovulation and fertilization.[2]

Clinical presentation
Implantation bleeding is characterized by scant pink or brownish discharge. It is not similar in volume or duration to typical menses. Most women experience no symptoms at the time of implantation, whereas others experience mild cramps or brief spotting.[2] The bleeding might be related temporally to implantation, but there is no clear evidence to support this concept.

Diagnosis and management
The differential diagnosis for vaginal bleeding during early pregnancy is broad. It includes spontaneous abortion, ectopic pregnancy, SH, HP, and anembryonic pregnancy.[3] Once these diagnoses have been ruled out, the management is expectant.

SH

Definition
SH occurs when the chorionic plate partially detaches from the underlying decidua of a normal ovum. It accounts for approximately 18% of all cases of bleeding during the first trimester.[4] Its size and location determine its effect on the pregnancy.

Clinical presentation
Patients may present with vaginal bleeding and abdominal pain. The differential diagnosis is initially broad. It includes spontaneous abortion, ectopic pregnancy, HP, and anembryonic pregnancy.[3]

Diagnosis and management
Ultrasonography is the ideal study to diagnose SH. It shows a normal gestational sac surrounded by a sonolucent gap between the chorion and the decidua. Initially, efforts should be directed at determining the health of the embryo by measuring the fetal heart rate. A rate less than 85 beats/min suggests a poor prognosis.[5] The location, size, and volume of the SH should also be noted. If the hematoma is found at the implantation site, it likely interrupts the maternal-embryonic exchange and therefore portends a poor prognosis. A large hematoma may fully separate the gestational sac from the endometrium, leading to spontaneous abortion. A hematoma of less than one-quarter of the gestation sac area is associated with a good prognosis.[5]

The management of SH is expectant. Either the hematoma is reabsorbed gradually, allowing the pregnancy to proceed to term, or its volume increases until it separates the gestational sac from the endometrium, leading to the demise of the embryo.[1,4] Patients should be advised to avoid activities that may induce uterine contractions or infection, such as intercourse, heavy lifting, douching, and tampon use. Avoidance of these activities is collectively known as pelvic rest.[1]

Ectopic Pregnancy

Definition
Ectopic pregnancy refers to the implantation of a fertilized ovum outside the uterine cavity.[6–8] It occurs in 2% of pregnancies and is the leading cause of first-trimester maternal death.[6] Risk factors for ectopic pregnancy include a previous ectopic

pregnancy, previous tubal surgery (including tubal ligation), tubal disease (previous sexually transmitted diseases and pelvic inflammatory disease), smoking, and current use of an intrauterine device.[9]

Clinical presentation

The clinical presentation differs depending on the timing of presentation: unruptured versus ruptured ectopic pregnancy. In unruptured cases, patients may present with nonspecific symptoms such as abdominal pain or cramping, light (bright or dark) vaginal bleeding, or both. Some women report a delayed menstrual period and most do not know they are pregnant.[7] These patients typically present with stable vital signs. The classic triad of amenorrhea, abdominal pain, and vaginal bleeding rarely present together. A study that reviewed 147 cases of ectopic pregnancy revealed that the most common presenting symptoms were abdominal pain (98%), amenorrhea (74%), and irregular vaginal bleeding (56%). The most common physical findings were abdominal tenderness (97%) and adnexal tenderness (98%).[10] Patients with ruptured ectopic pregnancies may present with signs of shock, including hypotension and tachycardia. Abdominal guarding, rigidity, or rebound tenderness may also be present. Like any other unstable patient, these patients need to be resuscitated emergently.[8]

Diagnosis and management

To prevent morbidity and mortality, early diagnosis of ectopic pregnancy is essential. Obtaining a serum human chorionic gonadotropin (hCG) level and a transvaginal ultra-sonography (TVUS) study are key elements of the initial workup. In the stable patient, the initial goal is to determine if the patient has an intrauterine pregnancy. Although an intrauterine pregnancy virtually rules out an ectopic pregnancy, the incidence of heterotopic pregnancies ranges from 1 in 30,000 in spontaneous conceptions to as high as 1 in 100 in assisted conceptions.[11]

TVUS can identify intrauterine pregnancies with nearly 100% accuracy at 5.5 weeks' gestation.[12] The first sonographic finding of an intrauterine pregnancy, at 4.5 to 5 weeks of gestation, is the presence of double echogenic rings around the gestational sac, also known as the double decidual sign. The next finding, at 5 to 6 weeks of gestation, is the yolk sac. Later, at 5.5 to 6 weeks of gestation, the fetal pole and cardiac activity can be detected.[8,13] When the weeks of presumed gestation are unknown, the serum hCG level can be used to indicate whether an intrauterine pregnancy should be visualized: a value within the discriminatory zone (1500–2500 mIU/mL) suggests that detection should be possible. An ectopic pregnancy should be highly suspected if the serum hCG level has reached the discriminatory zone and an intrauterine pregnancy cannot be visualized. Ideally, an ectopic pregnancy should be diagnosed by visualization of an extrauterine (adnexal) mass rather than the absence of an intrauterine pregnancy[6]; however, ectopic pregnancies are not always visualized on ultrasonography. Please see the article on ultrasound in pregnancy by Hsu and Euerle elsewhere in this issue for additional information.

Once an unruptured ectopic pregnancy has been confirmed, the treatment can be medical or surgical. The mainstay of medical treatment is methotrexate. The absolute indications for its administration are hemodynamic stability without signs of bleeding or hemoperitoneum, the patient's desire for future fertility, potential for significant adverse reactions to general anesthesia, no contraindication to methotrexate administration, and her ability to return for follow-up care. Relative indications include an unruptured mass less than 3.5 cm at its greatest dimension, no fetal cardiac activity, and a serum hCG level less than a predetermined value of 6 to 15,000 mIU/mL depending on institutional laboratory standards.[14] The absolute contraindications for use of methotrexate are summarized in **Box 1**. Relative contraindications include gestational sac greater than 3.5 cm at its greatest dimension and fetal cardiac activity.[14]

Many methotrexate protocols are available, but there is no consensus as to which should be used. Administration of this drug should be started in consultation with an obstetrician/gynecologist. With close follow-up, the patient's serum hCG level can be monitored to ensure that it decreases to zero.[15] Patients should understand that they remain at risk of rupture while being treated with methotrexate. The success rate of methotrexate has been linked to many factors, but it seems that the serum hCG level is the best single predictive factor.[16] For instance, patients with a serum hCG concentration less than 5000 mIU/mL have the greatest success. Levels between 5000 and 9999 mIU/mL have failure rates of 13%, and those with levels more than 15,000 mIU/mL have failure rates as high as 32%.[16] When medical treatment is not an option, surgical management includes laparoscopic salpingectomy or salpingostomy.

Patients who present to the emergency department with signs of a ruptured ectopic pregnancy (tachycardia, hypotension, and peritoneal signs) should be resuscitated immediately and taken to the operating room for emergent intervention.[6,17]

HP

Definition

An HP is the simultaneous occurrence of intrauterine and extrauterine pregnancies.[18] The incidence of HP varies significantly between spontaneous and assisted conception populations. In spontaneous conceptions with no risk factors, the incidence is 1 in 30,000. However, in assisted conception through in vitro fertilization, the incidence has been reported at 1 in 100 to 500. Other risk factors include the use of intrauterine devices, pelvic inflammatory disease, and tubal surgeries.[19]

Clinical presentation

The most common symptom of HP is abdominal pain. Most patients present emergently with signs and symptoms suggestive of a ruptured ectopic pregnancy. Most of these women are already aware that they are carrying an intrauterine pregnancy.[11]

Diagnosis and management

Early in pregnancy, the diagnosis of HP can be challenging, given that the sensitivity of transvaginal sonography to detect HP is only 56% at 5 to 6 weeks.[11] An extrauterine

---

Box 1
Absolute contraindications to methotrexate administration

Breastfeeding

Immunodeficiency

Abnormal creatinine level (>1.3 mg/dL)

Abnormal aspartate aminotransferase (more than twice the normal value)

Alcoholism or liver disease

Preexisting blood disorders

Peptic ulcer disease

Pulmonary disease

Known sensitivity to methotrexate

pregnancy often goes unnoticed when an intrauterine pregnancy has been identified. The diagnosis becomes more obvious with sonographic findings such as hemosalpinx or hemoperitoneum, especially if they are accompanied by signs and symptoms of hemodynamic instability. Because of the increasing use of assisted-conception techniques, physicians must always include heterotopic pregnancies in their differential diagnosis in this patient population. The management of HP aims to eliminate the ectopic pregnancy and maintain the intrauterine pregnancy. If the ectopic pregnancy is detected early, management can include aspiration and instillation of potassium chloride or prostaglandin into the gestational sac. Otherwise, using a laparoscopic approach, the ectopic pregnancy can be removed without disrupting the intrauterine pregnancy.[11,19,20]

Spontaneous Abortion (Miscarriage)

Definition
Approximately 15% of pregnancies are miscarried. Eighty percent of all miscarriages occur before the 12th week. A review of the literature suggests that these numbers may be even higher because many women miscarry before they know that they are pregnant. Increasing maternal age increases the risk of miscarriage.[21] Miscarriages can progress from threatened miscarriage to inevitable miscarriage to complete miscarriage.

Clinical presentation, diagnosis, and management
Patients who are less than 20 weeks pregnant and present with vaginal bleeding and no cervical dilation or effacement are experiencing a threatened miscarriage. Vaginal bleeding can range from spotting to severe bleeding lasting from hours to days. Some patients experience abdominal cramping, but others do not.[21] A pelvic examination reveals a closed internal cervical os with no tissue passage. Pelvic ultrasonography may show a gestation sac as early as 5.5 weeks of gestation. Some of the characteristics of impending miscarriage are an abnormal gestational sac size, a small embryo for the period of gestation, and a slow fetal heart rate.[22] The diagnosis of a threatened miscarriage and the possible miscarriage process should be delivered to the patient carefully, because this is likely to be an emotionally charged conversation. Patients should see an obstetrician within 3 days after the emergency department evaluation for serial serum hCG measurements.[1] They should return to the emergency department if they experience increased vaginal bleeding, light-headedness, fever, or abdominal pain.

Patients experiencing inevitable miscarriages have an open cervical os with or without evidence of tissue passage on pelvic examination. These patients miscarry spontaneously. Vaginal bleeding accompanied by abdominal cramping should be expected. Gentle removal of products of conception found at the os may facilitate completion of the miscarriage.[1] These patients must be evaluated by an obstetrician for possible uterine curettage.

Patients with complete miscarriage have experienced total expulsion of products of conception and have no additional symptoms. Pelvic examination usually reveals a closed cervical os. Ultrasonography confirms the diagnosis by showing an empty uterus.[1,21] If the diagnosis is certain, no additional emergent interventions are necessary. However, patients should be encouraged to pursue outpatient follow-up with an obstetrician.

Incomplete miscarriage is similar to complete miscarriage in that all symptoms seem to have resolved. A pelvic examination shows a closed cervical os. However, an ultrasonographic examination reveals retained fetal or placental tissue in the uterus.[22,23] These patients should be evaluated promptly by an obstetrician for uterine dilation and curettage to decrease the chance of recurrent bleeding and infection.[21]

Any of these types of miscarriage can lead to an intrauterine infection, called a septic miscarriage. Risk factors include elective termination with poor aseptic techniques or inadequate evacuation of the uterus, use of intrauterine devices, infection with the human immunodeficiency virus, and diabetes.[1,20] Patients present with fever and lower abdominal pain. Appropriate laboratory tests include a complete blood cell count and blood and cervical cultures. Antibiotic treatment should include coverage for gram-positive and gram-negative anaerobic and aerobic organisms. Emergent obstetric consultation should be obtained for dilation and curettage.

Anembryonic Pregnancy

Definition
An anembryonic pregnancy or blighted ovum occurs when a gestation sac develops without any embryonic structures.[24]

Clinical presentation
Patients may present with vaginal bleeding or abdominal pain.

Diagnosis and management
Anembryonic pregnancies are diagnosed by ultrasonography. Typically, ultrasonography shows a gestation sac greater than 13 mm in diameter without a yolk sac, a gestation sac greater than 18 mm in diameter without an embryonic pole, an empty sac beyond 38 days' gestation, or no interval growth over 1 week.[25] Management with misoprostol and uterine aspiration is effective.[26]

Rh Immune Globulin

An Rh-negative pregnant woman who is exposed to Rh-positive fetal blood is at risk for isoimmunization. Future exposures to Rh-positive antigen may result in the production of Rh immunoglobulin G (RhIG) antibodies, which can cause fetal morbidity (fetal anemia, erythroblastosis fetalis), and mortality.[27] Although the administration of RhIG has been shown to be effective in reducing maternal sensitization and fetal morbidity and mortality peripartum and during the third trimester,[28] its use during the first trimester remains controversial. There is little evidence to support the use of first-trimester RhIG; however, it has become standard of care as a result of expert opinion and extrapolation on experience with third-trimester fetomaternal hemorrhage.[29,30] The current recommendations by the American College of Obstetricians and Gynecologists state that all unsensitized Rh-negative pregnant women should be given RhIG within 72 hours of abortion. The recommended doses are 50 μg of RhIG before 12 weeks of gestation and 300 μg after 12 weeks of gestation.[27]

FIRST-TRIMESTER ABDOMINAL PAIN AND VOMITING
HG

Definition
HG occurs in 0.3% to 2% of pregnant women.[31] Although nausea and vomiting are nearly universal during pregnancy, HG is a condition characterized by persistent vomiting, weight loss of more than 5% (or 3 kg) of prepregnancy weight, ketonuria, electrolyte abnormalities (hypokalemia), and dehydration (high urine specific gravity).[32] The cause of HG remains unclear; however, many studies have linked it to levels of serum hCG and estradiol.[31] The theory suggests that hCG stimulates estrogen production from the ovary and that estrogen in turn induces nausea and vomiting.[32]

Furthermore, HG might be caused by products of placental metabolism, as shown by the fact that it occurs in molar pregnancies when a fetus is not present.[33]

Clinical presentation

HG can occur as early as the fifth week after the last menstrual period, but it peaks at 8 to 12 weeks. In most women, it resolves by 16 to 18 weeks.[34] If not treated properly, HG can lead to serious maternal complications. A rare but serious one is Wernicke encephalopathy, caused by thiamine (vitamin B_1) deficiency. The classic triad comprises ophthalmoplegia, gait ataxia, and confusion; however, the most common symptoms reported in practice are apathy and confusion.[31] This condition can occur as early as after 3 weeks of persistent vomiting. Patients with HG should not be treated with intravenous dextrose without thiamine because dextrose metabolism rapidly consumes any available thiamine, leading to acute encephalopathy.[32]

Diagnosis and management

It is important to determine the severity of dehydration and starvation in patients suspected of having HG. Laboratory testing includes urinalysis (ketones), basic metabolic panel (electrolyte abnormalities, blood urea nitrogen, and creatinine), liver enzymes, bilirubin, lipase, and thyroid-stimulating hormone (TSH) (suppressed TSH or increase in free thyroxine).[31,32,34] Abnormalities in these parameters improve with resolution of HG without additional interventions.[35] The treatment of HG is supportive and geared toward relief of symptoms.[34] In the acute setting, patients should be rehydrated with intravenous fluids and given intravenous antiemetics. There is limited evidence from trials to guide the choice of antiemetic drugs for HG.[33] However, current recommendations include intravenous metoclopramide or promethazine as first-line agents and methylprednisolone (only after 10 weeks' gestation) or ondansetron as second-line agent.[32] In practice, combination therapy is commonly used. Patients with HG might also benefit from vitamin B_6, which has been shown in randomized, placebo-controlled trials to be effective in the treatment of nausea and vomiting in pregnancy.[32]

GTD: Hydatidiform Mole and Gestational Trophoblastic Neoplasia

GTD is a spectrum of disease processes that originate from the placenta. It has 4 clinicopathologic forms: hydatidiform mole (complete and partial), invasive mole, choriocarcinoma, and placental site trophoblastic tumor. Because of their ability to progress to invasive and metastatic disease, the last 3 have been termed gestational trophoblastic neoplasia (GTN).[36]

Hydatidiform mole

Definition A hydatidiform mole can be complete or partial. Complete molar pregnancies are fully derived from the paternal genome. They arise from reduplication of the haploid genome of the sperm. The most common karyotype is 46XX. Partial molar pregnancies have a triploid karyotype. These karyotypes usually form after fertilization of a normal ovum by 2 sperm. The most common karyotype is 69XXX (23 chromosomes of maternal origin and 46 of paternal origin).[37,38] In the United States, hydatidiform moles are observed in approximately 1 in 600 therapeutic abortions and 1 in 1000 to 1200 pregnancies.[39]

Clinical presentation In the past, complete hydatidiform moles were usually diagnosed during the second trimester. The classic signs and symptoms included excessive uterine size, hyperemesis, anemia, toxemia, hyperthyroidism, and respiratory failure. Over the past few decades, as a result of the development of sensitive tests for detection of hCG and the wide use of ultrasonography, detection usually occurs during the first trimester, often before any of the classic symptoms appear.[40] Partial hydatidiform moles, on the other hand, present with the signs and symptoms of missed or incomplete abortion, such as vaginal bleeding and uterine size that is small or appropriate for the reported gestational age.[40,41]

Diagnosis and management Ultrasonography and serum hCG levels are used to diagnose hydatidiform molar pregnancies. The chorionic villi of complete moles show diffuse hydropic swelling, which appears as a distinct ultrasonographic pattern characterized by multiple echoes within the placenta and no associated fetus. In the case of partial moles, ultrasonography may show focal cystic spaces within the placenta as well as an increase in the transverse diameter of the gestation sac.[36] The hCG level in approximately 50% of women before evacuation of a complete mole is greater than 100,000 mIU/mL. However, partial moles do not typically present with such high levels of hCG. Only 10% of patients have a level greater than 100,000 mIU/mL at the time of diagnosis. The management of both entities includes surgical evacuation followed by close monitoring of the hCG level after evacuation.

GTN

After the evacuation of a hydatidiform mole, patients' hCG levels must be followed to monitor them for trophoblastic sequelae (invasive mole or choriocarcinoma), which develop in 15% to 20% of women with complete mole and 1% to 5% with partial mole. Invasive mole is a benign tumor that results from myometrial invasion of a hydatidiform mole. It usually metastasizes to the lungs or vagina. It is frequently treated with chemotherapy. Choriocarcinoma is a malignant disease that occurs via direct invasion of the myometrium and progression to widely disseminated vascular invasion to lungs, vagina, brain, and liver.[36,42] These tumors are perfused by fragile vessels, so metastases are often hemorrhagic. Patients can present emergently with signs and symptoms of bleeding from metastases, such as hemoptysis, intraperitoneal bleeding, and acute neurologic deficits. Treatment typically requires a combination of chemotherapy, radiation, and surgical interventions.[42]

FIRST-TRIMESTER ABDOMINAL PAIN
Round Ligament Syndrome

Definition
Pelvic and back pain are common in pregnancy and their incidence tends to increase as the pregnancy progresses. Round ligament syndrome is pain related to normal changes that occur as the uterus increases in size during pregnancy. The round ligament suspends the uterus in place. As the uterus increases in size and weight, these ligaments become long and thin and, as they stretch, they cause pain.[43,44]

Clinical presentation
Patients with round ligament syndrome present with the complaint of pelvic pain and low back pain. Ligament spasms can trigger severe sharp pain. There is a predilection for worse symptoms on the right side, because the uterus tends to turn to the right. This pain can be debilitating, affecting the patient's activities of daily living, including the ability to work. The pain is often worse at night and it may occur suddenly when the patient turns while sleeping.[44]

Diagnosis and management
A thorough history and physical examination must be performed on these patients, because abdominal/pelvic pain in a pregnant woman can have many more dangerous causes. Interventions such as special pregnancy exercises, frequent rest, hot and cold

compresses, supportive belts, acupuncture, and yoga have been suggested. A 2008 Cochrane review set out to assess the effects of interventions for preventing and treating back and pelvic pain in pregnancy. No studies were found regarding their prevention. However, the investigators reviewed 8 trials, involving 1305 participants, which examined the effects of various pregnancy-specific exercises, physiotherapy programs, acupuncture, and special pillows. The investigators found that specifically tailored strengthening exercises, sitting pelvic-tilt exercise regimens, and water gymnastics had positive effects. Furthermore, acupuncture seemed to be more effective than physiotherapy.[43]

SUMMARY

The emergency physician must be skilled at evaluating and managing first-trimester vaginal bleeding and abdominal pain. Because some of the complications of these presentations can be life-threatening, the old emergency medicine teaching, "Assume that every woman of childbearing age is pregnant," rings ever more true. This article discusses the presentation and diagnosis of implantation bleeding, SH, spontaneous abortion, ectopic pregnancy, HP, anembryonic pregnancy, HG, GTD, and round ligament syndrome and current guidelines for their treatment. As we care for these patients, it is important to take time and recognize that these diagnoses are emotionally charged and often affect the patient's future fertility.

REFERENCES

1. Deutchman M, Tubay AT, Turok D. First trimester bleeding. Am Fam Physician 2009;79:985–94.
2. Harville EW, Wilcox AJ, Baird DD, et al. Vaginal bleeding in very early pregnancy. Hum Reprod 2003;18:1944–7.
3. Condous G. The management of early pregnancy complications. Best Pract Res Clin Obstet Gynaecol 2004;18:37–57.
4. Pelinescu-Onciul D. Subchorionic hemorrhage treatment with dydrogesterone. Gynecol Endocrinol 2007;23(Suppl 1):77–81.
5. Norman SM, Odibo AO, Macones GA, et al. Ultrasound-detected subchorionic hemorrhage and the obstetric implications. Obstet Gynecol 2010;116:311–5.
6. Nama V, Manyonda I. Tubal ectopic pregnancy: diagnosis and management. Arch Gynecol Obstet 2009;279:443–53.
7. Barnhart KT. Clinical practice: ectopic pregnancy. N Engl J Med 2009;361: 379–87.
8. Mukul LV, Teal SB. Current management of ectopic pregnancy. Obstet Gynecol Clin North Am 2007;34:403–19.
9. Ankum WM, Mol BW, Van der Veen F, et al. Risk factors for ectopic pregnancy: a meta-analysis. Fertil Steril 1996;65:1093–9.
10. Alsuleiman SA, Grimes EM. Ectopic pregnancy: a review of 147 cases. J Reprod Med 1982;27:101–6.
11. Hassani KI, Bouazzaoui AE, Khatouf M, et al. Heterotopic pregnancy: a diagnosis we should suspect more often. J Emerg Trauma Shock 2010;3:304.
12. Gracia CR, Barnhart KT. Diagnosing ectopic pregnancy: decision analysis comparing six strategies. Obstet Gynecol 2001;97:464–70.
13. Bradley WG, Fiske CE, Filly RA. The double sac sign of early intrauterine pregnancy: use in exclusion of ectopic pregnancy. Radiology 1982;143:223–6.
14. ACOG practice bulletin. Medical management of tubal pregnancy. Number 3, December 1998. Clinical management guidelines for obstetrician-gynecologists.

American College of Obstetricians and Gynecologists. Int J Gynaecol Obstet 1999; 65:97–103.

15. Sowter MC, Farquhar CM. Ectopic pregnancy: an update. Curr Opin Obstet Gynecol 2004;16:289–93.

16. Lipscomb GH, McCord ML, Stovall TG, et al. Predictors of success of methotrexate treatment in women with tubal ectopic pregnancies. N Engl J Med 1999;341:1974–8.

17. Jurkovic D, Wilkinson H. Diagnosis and management of ectopic pregnancy. BMJ 2011;342:d3397.

18. Cappell MS, Friedel D. Abdominal pain during pregnancy. Gastroenterol Clin North Am 2003;32:1–58.

19. Anastasakis E, Jetti A, Macara L, et al. A case of heterotopic pregnancy in the absence of risk factors: a brief literature review. Fetal Diagn Ther 2007;22:285–8.

20. Woodfield CA, Lazarus E, Chen KC, et al. Abdominal pain in pregnancy: diagnoses and imaging unique to pregnancy–review. AJR Am J Roentgenol 2010; 194:WS14–30.

21. Coppola PT, Coppola M. Vaginal bleeding in the first 20 weeks of pregnancy. Emerg Med Clin North Am 2003;21:667–77.

22. Paspulati RM, Bhatt S, Nour SG. Sonographic evaluation of first-trimester bleeding. Radiol Clin North Am 2004;42:297–314.

23. Dighe M, Cuevas C, Moshiri M, et al. Sonography in first trimester bleeding. J Clin Ultrasound 2008;36:352–66.

24. Prine LW, MacNaughton H. Office management of early pregnancy loss. Am Fam Physician 2011;84:75–82.

25. Cho FN, Chen SN, Tai MH, et al. The quality and size of yolk sac in early pregnancy loss. Aust N Z J Obstet Gynaecol 2006;46:413–8.

26. Odeh M, Tendler R, Kais M, et al. Gestational sac volume in missed abortion and anembryonic pregnancy compared to normal pregnancy. J Clin Ultrasound 2010;38:367–71.

27. ACOG practice bulletin. Prevention of Rh D alloimmunization. Number 4, May 1999 (replaces educational bulletin number 147, October 1990). Clinical management guidelines for obstetrician-gynecologists. American College of Obstetrics and Gynecology. Int J Gynaecol Obstet 1999;66:63–70.

28. Urbaniak SJ. The scientific basis of antenatal prophylaxis. Br J Obstet Gynaecol 1998;105(Suppl 18):11–8.

29. Jabara S, Barnhart KT. Is Rh immune globulin needed in early first-trimester abortion? A review. Am J Obstet Gynecol 2003;188:623–7.

30. Hannafin B, Lovecchio F, Blackburn P. Do Rh-negative women with first trimester spontaneous abortions need Rh immune globulin? Am J Emerg Med 2006;24:487–9.

31. Goodwin TM. Hyperemesis gravidarum. Obstet Gynecol Clin North Am 2008;35:401–17.

32. Niebyl JR. Clinical practice. Nausea and vomiting in pregnancy. N Engl J Med 2010;363:1544–50.

33. Tan PC, Omar SZ. Contemporary approaches to hyperemesis during pregnancy. Curr Opin Obstet Gynecol 2011;23:87–93.

34. Sonkusare S. The clinical management of hyperemesis gravidarum. Arch Gynecol Obstet 2011;283:1183–92.

35. Jarvis S, Nelson-Piercy C. Management of nausea and vomiting in pregnancy. BMJ 2011;342:d3606.

36. Lurain JR. Gestational trophoblastic disease I: epidemiology, pathology, clinical presentation and diagnosis of gestational trophoblastic disease, and management of hydatidiform mole. Am J Obstet Gynecol 2010;203:531–9.

37. Hurteau JA. Gestational trophoblastic disease: management of hydatidiform mole. Clin Obstet Gynecol 2003;46:557–69.
38. Seckl MJ, Sebire NJ, Berkowitz RS. Gestational trophoblastic disease. Lancet 2010;376:717–29.
39. Soper JT. Gestational trophoblastic disease. Obstet Gynecol 2006;108:176–87.
40. Berkowitz RS, Goldstein DP. Clinical practice. molar pregnancy. N Engl J Med 2009;360:1639–45.
41. Sebire NJ, Seckl MJ. Gestational trophoblastic disease: current management of hydatidiform mole. BMJ 2008;337:a1193.
42. Berkowitz RS, Goldstein DP. Current management of gestational trophoblastic diseases. Gynecol Oncol 2009;112:654–62.
43. Pennick VE, Young G. Interventions for preventing and treating pelvic and back pain in pregnancy. Cochrane Database Syst Rev 2007;(2):CD001139.
44. Malmqvist S, Kjaermann I, Andersen K, et al. Prevalence of low back and pelvic pain during pregnancy in a Norwegian population. J Manipulative Physiol Ther 2012;35:272–8.

Ultrasound in Pregnancy

Sam Hsu, MD, RDMS*, Brian D. Euerle, MD, RDMS

KEYWORDS

- Ultrasound • Pregnancy • Ectopic pregnancy • Heterotopic pregnancy
- Fetal heart rate • Fetal gestational age

KEY POINTS

- Transabdominal ultrasound, which uses a curvilinear 3- to 6-MHz probe, should be attempted initially in all cases, even in early pregnancy, because it provides a good overview of the entire abdomen including the pelvis. It can be used throughout all stages of pregnancy.
- Transvaginal ultrasound uses a 6- to 10-MHz intracavitary probe, the transducer of which is inserted into the anterior fornix. Because this technique uses a higher-frequency transducer, it provides a higher-resolution image, which is especially useful during the earliest stages of pregnancy.
- Ultrasound can be used to rapidly estimate fetal gestational age. Different measurements are used depending on the stage of the pregnancy and include mean sac diameter (earliest stage), crown-rump length, biparietal diameter, and femur length.
- Identifying an intrauterine pregnancy dramatically lowers the possibility of an ectopic pregnancy. However, because of the concern for heterotopic pregnancy, the overall clinical presentation of the patient must be kept in mind.

INTRODUCTION

Obstetric emergencies are a significant part of the practice of emergency medicine, and their management can be quite challenging. To successfully evaluate and treat these patients, emergency physicians must use all the tools at their disposal. One of the most important tools is point-of-care ultrasound. Ultrasound is the ideal imaging modality to use in the pregnant patient; it lacks ionizing radiation and presents minimal risk to the mother and the developing fetus. The concept of point-of-care, or bedside, ultrasound emphasizes that the providers caring for patients perform the ultrasound themselves, at the bedside, rather than sending the patient to another location,

Disclosures: The authors have no financial or other relationships that could impact the content of this article.
Department of Emergency Medicine, University of Maryland School of Medicine, 110 South Paca Street, Sixth Floor, Suite 200, Baltimore, MD 21201, USA
* Corresponding author.
E-mail address: shsu@umem.org

possibly distant from the emergency department (ED), to have the ultrasound performed by another provider. This approach allows the emergency physician to get immediate ultrasound results, while keeping patients in the ED, where they can be monitored and resuscitated if needed. This approach decreases patient time in the ED.[1]

Ultrasound has two broad areas of application in pregnant patients in the ED. The first is that it can provide information that is useful in all pregnant patients, including gestational age. Many patients presenting to the ED are unsure of their last menstrual period or the stage of their pregnancy. By using bedside ultrasound early in the evaluation, the emergency physician can obtain an estimated gestational age, which allows rapid refinement of what diagnoses should be considered in that particular patient. Many EDs triage patients above a certain gestational age directly to the hospital obstetric or labor and delivery unit for evaluation and management, and ultrasound is the ideal tool for this decision-making process. Fetal heart rate is another measurement that can be obtained easily in most pregnant patients in the ED.

The second broad area of use of ultrasound is in assessment of patients suspected of having an ectopic pregnancy (EP). The mortality rate associated with EP has improved markedly, yet it remains the leading cause of death in the first trimester of pregnancy.[2] The patient with an EP can present to the ED in a variety of states, ranging from well appearing with no or minimal complaints to critically ill in hemorrhagic shock or cardiac arrest. Patients at either end of this spectrum should be evaluated in a rapid and efficient manner, and bedside ultrasound can play a large role.

INDICATIONS

Indications for ultrasound in pregnancy include to confirm that a patient is pregnant, to estimate gestational age, to determine fetal heart rate, to evaluate a patient suspected of having an EP, and to evaluate a patient with suspected fetal demise.

CONTRAINDICATIONS

Ultrasound in a patient that needs to go immediately to the operating room is contraindicated if the performance of the ultrasound would delay that process.

TECHNIQUE

Obstetric ultrasound can be done with either a transabdominal (TA) or transvaginal (TV) approach. Each offers its own advantages and disadvantages, and there are differences in the equipment and approach used by each.

Equipment

A curvilinear 3- to 6-MHz probe is part of most ultrasound systems and the probe of choice for imaging the pregnant patient. It is used to obtain TA views of the uterus. It provides a broad field of view and has good penetration to the uterus. Adequate images may not be possible for two main reasons: very early pregnancy and retroverted or retroflexed uterus. In early pregnancy, the gestational structures may be too small or too deep for the probe to image. With a retroverted or retroflexed uterus, bowel occupies the space anterior to the uterus, making it difficult, if not impossible, to image.

When the TA approach fails, or if additional information is desired, a TV probe is necessary. TV probes are higher frequency, 6 to 10 MHz, compared with TA probes, so they provide a more detailed image. This allows visualization of gestational anatomy up to a week earlier than a TA approach. The main disadvantage of TV probes, besides being invasive, is that it can be difficult to visualize the anatomic relationships of organs because all the structures are seen in close-up. The TV approach is rarely needed beyond 8 weeks' gestation because structures are large enough to be imaged adequately by the TA approach.

Acoustic gel is needed for either approach. A gel warmer is helpful for patient comfort but is rarely available in the ED. In addition, the TV probe needs a cover, which can be specially designed for the probe or a sterile glove can be used.

Consideration must also be given to equipment to clean the TV probe between uses. A TV probe requires high-level disinfection because of the possibility of leakage of the cover during use. The most common method is to immerse the probe in a glutaraldehyde (Cidex) solution. Probe manufacturers list compatible disinfection solutions for their specific probes, and the American Institute of Ultrasound in Medicine has published guidelines on probe cleaning.[3]

Preparation

Patient preparation differs in the TA and TV approaches. With TA scanning, the presence of a full urinary bladder is helpful because it acts as an acoustic window and improves the images that are obtained.[4] Historically, the bladder was filled before an ultrasound examination to displace bowel from the imaging plane; however, a full bladder is not a requirement and TA scanning need not be delayed if the bladder is empty.[5] The opposite situation exists during TV scanning: a full bladder can be detrimental because it can displace the uterus posteriorly, potentially out of the limited field of view of the TV probe. In addition, the patient can experience additional discomfort during TV scanning with the bladder full. Therefore, the patient should be instructed to empty her bladder before TV scanning. These recommendations work well with the common pattern of performing TA ultrasound first. The patient can then empty her bladder, and undergo TV ultrasound.

Patient Positioning

The ideal patient position depends on the type of scanning that is being done. For TA scanning, the patient is placed in the supine position. When performing TA obstetric scanning, the physician may elect to use the TA probe to look elsewhere in the abdomen, specifically at Morison pouch in the right upper quadrant, because free fluid (blood) from a leaking or ruptured EP is likely to collect there. There have been some reports that placing a patient in the Trendelenburg position increases the sensitivity of detection of free fluid in the Morison pouch view.[6] Depending on the clinical situation, the physician may decide to place the patient in Trendelenburg after the pelvic portion of the examination has been completed, and then examine Morison pouch.

TV scanning is best accomplished with the patient in the lithotomy position, on a stretcher that is equipped with foot stirrups and typically used for performing pelvic examinations. This position, which places the patient's buttocks at the end of the stretcher, is essential because it allows the handle of the TV probe to be moved freely in any direction. Many physicians find it convenient and time effective to perform a manual pelvic examination first, immediately followed by TV ultrasound, keeping the patient in the same lithotomy position.

Transabdominal

A TA approach should be attempted initially in all cases, even in early pregnancy. It provides a good overview of the pelvis, and if adequate images are obtained, in some circumstances it may negate the need for the TV approach.[7] The easiest method of finding the uterus is to identify the bladder first. To do this, orient the probe longitudinally and place it immediately cephalad to the pubis symphysis. The probe should then be directed caudally so that the beam is pointed into the pelvis. The bladder is easily identified as an anechoic structure within the pelvis. The uterus is reliably found cephalad and deep to the bladder. On the ultrasound display, the uterus appears to the left of the bladder (**Fig. 1**). Usually, the only solid structures in the pelvis are the gynecologic organs and the bladder, so if it is not bowel or bladder, it is likely to be the uterus.

A full bladder is not needed to obtain usable images. If the bladder is full, it can help to displace bowel from the imaging plane, but gentle pressure with the probe often suffices to displace the bowel and obtain a view. If there is difficulty identifying the uterus, sweep the probe left to right. The uterus is not always in the midline. After the uterus is identified, look for signs of an intrauterine gestation. The probe may need to be rotated to obtain the best view of gestational structures.

Transvaginal

The probe is prepared by first placing gel on it, placing a probe cover, and then putting more gel over the cover. Insert the probe vaginally and direct it anteriorly. The goal is to place the probe in the anterior fornix against the cervix. A common error is directing the probe straight along the vaginal canal and placing it in the posterior fornix. When this happens, only bowel is visible, leading to frustrated searches for the uterus. If the uterus is retroflexed, the only way to visualize it is deliberate probe placement in the posterior fornix.

The TV probe should be oriented initially so that the indicator is pointed to the ceiling. This gives a sagittal image of the uterus (**Fig. 2**). The probe should be swept left to right to identify a gestational sac. When found, the probe can be rotated to obtain the best view of the gestational anatomy.

To visualize the cervix and posterior cul-de-sac, orient the probe sagittally and direct the beam posteriorly by lifting the probe handle (**Fig. 3**). To visualize the adnexa, orient the probe coronally by rotating it counterclockwise so that the indicator is toward the patient's right. This produces a cross-sectional image of the uterus. Direct the beam to either the right or left, keeping the uterus in view to maintain orientation, then sweep the beam anterior to posterior by moving the handle up and down. The

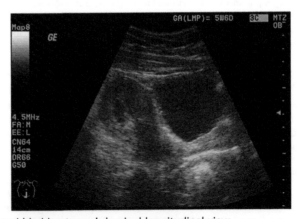

Fig. 1. Uterus and bladder, transabdominal longitudinal view.

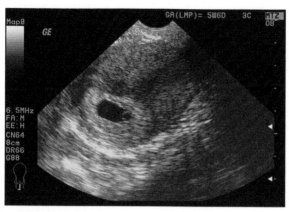

Fig. 2. Uterus, transvaginal sagittal view.

ovaries and adnexal mass are typically positioned medial to the external iliac vessels and lateral to the uterus (**Fig. 4**).

CLINICAL IMPLICATIONS
Normal Findings

First-trimester obstetric ultrasound is unique among the applications of emergency ultrasound in that normal anatomy changes with time. An understanding of developmental anatomy is essential to proper interpretation of the images.

During the first 4 weeks of gestation, the uterus appears very similar to the nonpregnant state. The endometrium is more echogenic than the myometrium during pregnancy. The opposing sides of the endometrium meet at a brightly echogenic stripe that makes the midline of the uterus easy to identify (**Fig. 5**).

The first anatomic sign of pregnancy is formation of the gestational sac. This is an intrauterine sac with a hyperechoic wall. The wall is composed of two layers that comprise the "double decidua": the decidua vera, which is derived from the endometrium, and the decidua capsularis, which is the wall surrounding the gestation (**Fig. 6**). The two layers are not always seen, but they become well delineated when

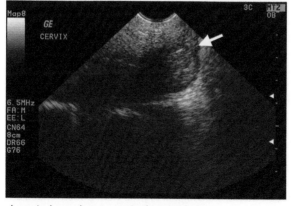

Fig. 3. Uterus and cervix (*arrow*), transvaginal sagittal view.

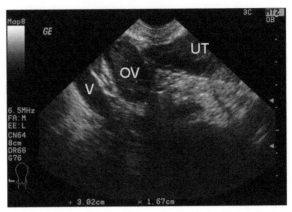

Fig. 4. Right adnexa, transvaginal coronal view. OV, ovary; UT, uterus; V, iliac vessels.

a subchorionic (implantation) hemorrhage is present, with blood occupying the potential space between the layers (**Fig. 7**). The gestational sac is visible on ultrasound between 4 and 5 weeks of gestation.

The second anatomic sign of pregnancy is the yolk sac. This is a hollow, hyperechoic circular structure found at the periphery of the gestational sac. The yolk sac typically appears during the fifth week of gestation (**Fig. 8**).

Soon after the appearance of the yolk sac, the embryo appears. It is often referred to as the "fetal pole" because of its appearance. It should be close to the yolk sac (**Fig. 9**). Very early in gestation, the characteristic flicker of a heartbeat can be seen near the yolk sac before the outline of the embryo is distinct. The heartbeat is easily seen by 6 weeks of gestation. The head bud appears distinct from the body in the seventh week of gestation and limbs in the eighth week. Around this time, the amniotic sac appears (**Fig. 10**). Beyond this period, the embryo transitions to a fetus and has a distinct baby-like appearance.

To confidently diagnose an intrauterine pregnancy (IUP), the emergency physician should visualize an intrauterine sac with at least a yolk sac. Although some practitioners are comfortable diagnosing an IUP based on an intrauterine sac that shows

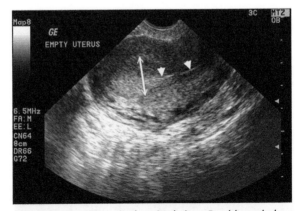

Fig. 5. Early gestation uterus, transvaginal sagittal view. *Double-ended arrow* indicates the endometrium; *arrowheads* indicate the uterine stripe.

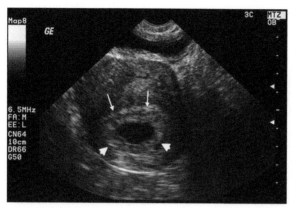

Fig. 6. Gestational sac with a double decidua. *Arrows* indicate the decidua vera; *arrowheads* indicate the decidua capsularis.

a clear double decidua, it is easy to mistake the various mimics as a gestational sac, most notably the pseudogestational sac of an EP.[5] The presence of a yolk sac ensures that the gestation is developing inside the uterus. Note that the fetal pole does not have to be present to make the distinction between an intrauterine and extrauterine pregnancy. The presence of the fetal pole is necessary only to determine the viability of the pregnancy.

Gestational Measurements

Two measurements are routinely obtained as part of an obstetric ultrasound: gestational age and fetal heart rate. The formulas are installed on most ultrasound machines and are accessible when the machine is placed in "OB mode."

Several methods can be used to measure gestational age. The choice is dictated by the developmental stage of the pregnancy. The most accurate and easiest to perform is crown-rump length. The main challenge is to obtain an image that shows the maximum length of the fetus. Before the fetus has limbs, the entire length of the fetal pole is measured. When limbs are present, only the distance from crown to rump is measured (**Fig. 11**). After the first trimester, the fetus is too large to view entirely in

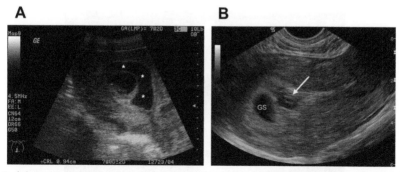

Fig. 7. (*A*) Gestational sac containing a fetal pole and yolk sac. *Asterisks* indicate a subchorionic hemorrhage separating the decidua vera and the decidua capsularis. (*B*) Gestational sac (GS). Subchorionic hemorrhage separating the decidua vera and the decidua capsularis (*arrow*).

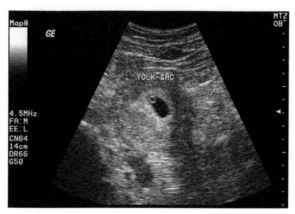

Fig. 8. Yolk sac located within a gestational sac.

a single image. In these cases, biparietal diameter and femur length are used to measure gestational age. The choice of which measurement to use is dictated by which part of the fetus is most clearly in view. To measure the biparietal diameter, a transverse view of the fetal head must be obtained. The central anterior-posterior fissure and thalamic nuclei must be depicted. The biparietal diameter is measured perpendicular to the central fissure and through the thalamic nuclei from the outer table of the proximal skull to the inner table of the distal skull (**Fig. 12**). The femur length is simply the length of the femur (**Fig. 13**). The main challenge is to obtain a true longitudinal view of the femur, because oblique views underestimate the true femur length and gestational age. For all these measurements, a menu option or "hotkey" needs to be selected before performing the measurement so that the correct calculation is performed.

Very early in pregnancy, there is no fetus to measure directly, so the mean sac diameter is measured. The mean sac diameter is an average of the length, width, and depth of the gestational sac. This measurement requires two orthogonal views of the sac, both showing the largest diameters possible. The depth is measured on one image, and the widths are measured on both images (**Fig. 14**). The ultrasound machine refers to a table that correlates mean sac diameter to gestational age. The tables have

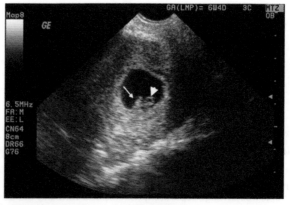

Fig. 9. Fetal pole (*arrow*) and yolk sac (*arrowhead*).

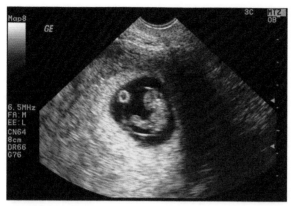

Fig. 10. Fetus surrounded by the amniotic sac.

a lower limit of mean sac diameter around 1 cm, which correlates to 5 weeks 5 days, so the gestational age cannot be measured accurately earlier than this point.

Fetal Heart Rate Determination

To measure the heart rate, activate M-mode and position the sampling line over the heartbeat. An undulating line representing cardiac motion appears on the M-mode tracing (**Fig. 15**). The heart rate is calculated by measuring the distance between one or two undulations. The specific measurement depends on the individual machine's set-up.

M-mode exposes the embryo to the same amount of ultrasonic energy as B-mode imaging. Doppler can highlight cardiac motion, but it exposes the embryo to significantly greater energies than B-mode or M-mode imaging and is generally unnecessary to locate cardiac activity. Because of the possibility of deleterious effects of high-energy ultrasound on growing embryos, emergency physicians should avoid routine use of Doppler modes.

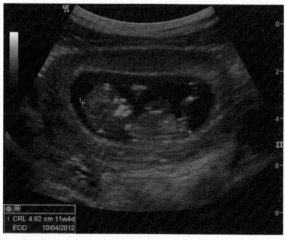

Fig. 11. Measurement of the crown-rump length.

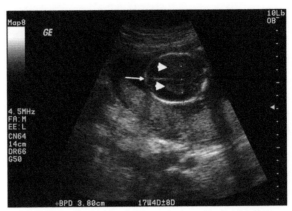

Fig. 12. Biparietal diameter measurement. The measurement is taken perpendicular to the central fissure (*arrow*) and through the thalamic nuclei (*arrowheads*).

Ectopic Pregnancy

The foremost question for a clinician faced with a symptomatic pregnant patient is: Does this patient have an EP? Ultrasound is part of the evaluation primarily to answer this question. In practical terms, when an IUP is identified, an EP is excluded. The assumption that underpins this interpretation is that heterotopic twins, concurrent IUP and EP, are a rare occurrence. The exact incidence is unknown because cases are not systematically reported. An often-cited estimate of 1 in 30,000 pregnancies was derived from the rates of dizygotic twins and EP in 1948.[8] Because the incidence of both has increased, current estimates are higher by an order of magnitude. A more recent calculation, based on the actual number of heterotopic pregnancies at two hospitals over a 4-year period, determined the incidence to be 1 in 3889 pregnancies.[9] The increase is caused among other factors by higher rates of pelvic inflammatory disease, invasive gynecologic procedures, and infertility treatments.[10] In vitro fertilization is a major risk factor, with 1 in 100 to 200 pregnancies resulting in heterotopic twins.[11] A history devoid of pelvic inflammatory disease, gynecologic surgery, and assisted pregnancy favors a very low likelihood of heterotopic pregnancy. However,

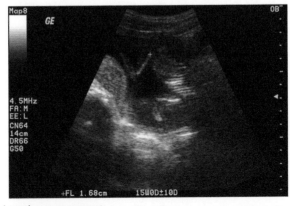

Fig. 13. Femur length measurement.

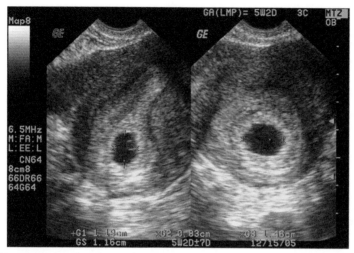

Fig. 14. Measurement of mean sac diameter.

patients without risk factors do develop heterotopic pregnancies; one review found that 29% of patients with heterotopic pregnancies had no risk factors.[12,13] Taking a history with specific attention to risk factors and carefully considering the severity of the clinical presentation minimizes the chance of overlooking a heterotopic twin pregnancy.

Fortunately, most pregnant patients presenting to the ED have an easily identifiable singleton IUP. When no IUP is present, then signs of EP must be sought. Ultrasound findings of EP fall into three categories: (1) definite extrauterine pregnancy, (2) highly suspicious for EP, and (3) the indeterminate scan.

A definite extrauterine pregnancy appears as a gestational sac with a yolk sac or fetal pole outside the boundaries of the uterus (**Fig. 16**). This finding is incontrovertible

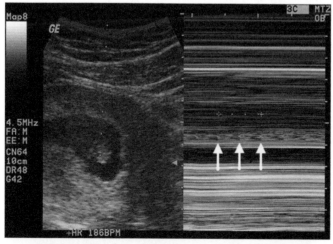

Fig. 15. Measurement of fetal heart rate using M-mode. *Arrows* indicate undulations, which each represent one cardiac cycle.

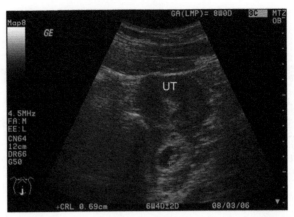

Fig. 16. Definite extrauterine pregnancy. The gestational sac containing a fetal pole is located outside the uterus (UT).

proof of an EP. Unfortunately, most EPs do not present with such certainty. Even ultrasounds performed and interpreted in the radiology department might not visualize an EP that is ultimately identified in the operating room. TV ultrasound has a sensitivity of 90.9% in detecting EP.[14] Bowel interference likely plays a factor in the low rates of visualization.

The category of "highly suspicious" for EP is broad and includes free fluid, adnexal masses, and tubal rings. The most sensitive and easiest sign to identify is free fluid around the uterus. Fluid can appear anechoic and homogeneous when it consists of serous fluid or recent hemorrhage, or "complex" and heterogeneous when composed of clotted blood and tissue. The likelihood of an EP rises with the amount of fluid present. Small amounts of free fluid are seen only in the posterior cul-de-sac and can be physiologic (**Fig. 17**). Moderate amounts of fluid can be seen surrounding the body of the uterus (**Fig. 18**). Large amounts of free fluid are seen distant from the uterus. If fluid is present around the liver (ie, a positive Morison pouch on focused assessment with sonography for trauma view) an EP is present until proved otherwise. The presence of echogenic fluid on ultrasound in a patient with a positive pregnancy

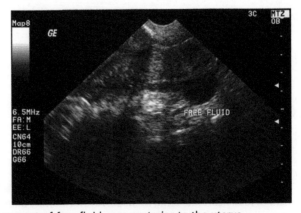

Fig. 17. Small amount of free fluid seen posterior to the uterus.

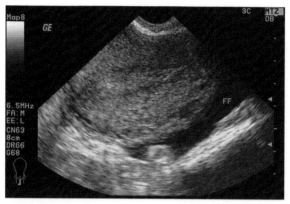

Fig. 18. Moderate amount of free fluid (FF) surrounding the uterus.

test has a positive predictive value of 86% to 93% for EP.[15] Somewhat counterintuitively, the finding of free fluid is not equivalent to rupture. Early in the course of an EP, blood can leak from the end of the fallopian tube before rupture. Free fluid could also occur because of ovarian cyst rupture, regardless of whether the pregnancy is an IUP or EP; however, the amount of fluid from a ruptured cyst should not be "large" or reach Morison pouch.

Adnexal masses are more difficult to find and not highly specific for EP. The differential diagnosis for adnexal masses includes complex or hemorrhagic ovarian cysts and neoplasms. Finding adnexal masses requires comfort with using the TV probe, familiarity with searching through the adnexal area, and experience in identifying ovaries and ovarian cysts. This requires a considerable amount of experience and is not a novice-level skill. A prerequisite to identifying adnexal masses is being able to distinguish them from normal ovaries. Ovaries are approximately 2 × 2 × 3 cm and may have small follicular cysts, giving them a "chocolate chip cookie" appearance (**Fig. 19**). A corpus luteum cyst may be present, appearing as a particularly large cyst (**Fig. 20**). Corpus luteum cysts can be simple or complex if hemorrhagic. Ovarian cysts should have very thin or no walls. A thick or echogenic wall should raise

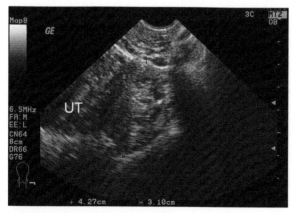

Fig. 19. Ovary, located adjacent to the uterus (UT).

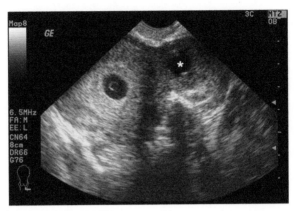

Fig. 20. Corpus luteum cyst (*asterisk*).

suspicion for a gestational sac. Ovaries have a relatively homogeneous appearance. Adnexal masses tend to be more complex, with variable echogenicity and irregular borders (**Fig. 21**). Adnexal masses were found in 61% of EPs in one report of emergency-physician-performed TV ultrasound.[16]

Tubal rings are the most difficult to find. They are gestational sacs within the fallopian tubes. Because they do not have a yolk sac or fetal pole within them, they are easily overlooked as a loop of bowel (**Fig. 22**). Tubal rings have been shown to have a sensitivity of 40% to 68% for EP.[17] Tubal rings enhance with Doppler, creating a "ring of fire" (**Fig. 23**). Because tubal rings can appear next to an ovary, distinguishing them from an exophytic corpus luteum cyst can be challenging. Even more confusing, corpus luteum cysts also enhance with Doppler (**Fig. 24**). One method to distinguish them is to apply pressure on the adnexal area with the probe and externally by hand. If the object in question moves independently from the ovary, it is extraovarian and suspicious for EP.[18] Because ovarian EPs are rare, ovarian cysts and masses are not likely to be an EP.

A pseudogestational sac is present in 10% of EPs.[19] Pseudogestational sacs are filled with blood and appear hypoechoic or anechoic (**Fig. 25**). Pseudogestational sacs are more irregular in shape and centrally located within the endometrial cavity,

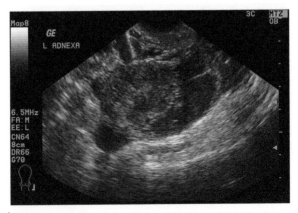

Fig. 21. Adnexal mass.

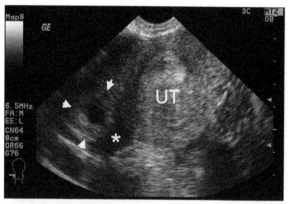

Fig. 22. Tubal ring. UT, uterus; asterisk, fluid.

whereas gestational sacs are more spherical and eccentrically located in the endometrium, but there is enough overlap in their features that they are easily confused for each other. For this reason, the safest practice is to avoid calling an intrauterine sac a gestational sac (ie, an IUP) until at least a yolk sac is inside it.

The final category of ultrasound finding is the indeterminate scan, which has the same appearance as a nongravid uterus. The management of these cases depends on the severity of the clinical presentation and whether there are any risk factors for EP. The quantitative human chorionic gonadotropin (HCG) level also plays a large role in the management decision. The HCG "discriminatory level," or "discriminatory zone," is the level above which an IUP should be visualized on TV ultrasound and is commonly reported to be between 1000 and 2000 mIU/mL. When no IUP is present and the HCG level is above the discriminatory level, most clinicians have a heightened suspicion for an EP. Unfortunately, the discriminatory level performs poorly as a dichotomous indicator for EP in this scenario. The differential diagnosis includes miscarriage and even normal early IUP. The quantitative HCG value can exceed the discriminatory level as early as the fourth week of gestation, when an indeterminate ultrasound is almost certain. Certainly, if there are "highly suspicious" findings on ultrasound, an HCG level above the discriminatory level provides compelling support for a diagnosis of EP. In cases of indeterminate scans, a single HCG measurement is

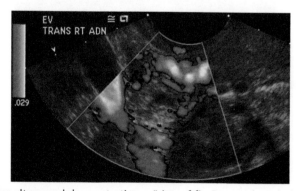

Fig. 23. Doppler ultrasound demonstrating a "ring of fire" around a tubal ring.

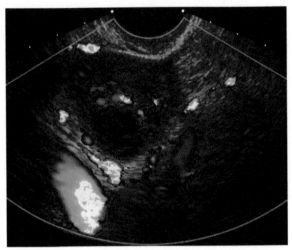

Fig. 24. Doppler ultrasound of a corpus luteum cyst simulating a "ring of fire."

not diagnostic in itself. Serial HCG measurements and ultrasounds are far more informative.

An unusual type of EP is the interstitial ectopic, which accounts for 2% to 4% of EPs.[20] Interstitial ectopics are located in the 1- to 2-cm segment of the fallopian tube that traverses the myometrium before terminating in the endometrial cavity. Interstitial EPs can appear to be IUPs because they are intrauterine yet confined within the fallopian tube and therefore have the same potential to rupture. Interstitial EP is suspected when less than 5 mm of myometrium surrounds the gestational sac. This criterion is not diagnostic: in one case report, a suspected interstitial EP based on it was later shown to be a normal IUP.[21] Cases in which the lateral superior part of the gestational sac appears to be outside the uterus are likely to be more specific for interstitial EP (**Fig. 26**).

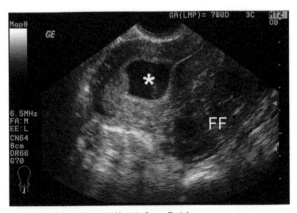

Fig. 25. Pseudogestational sac (*asterisk*). FF, free fluid.

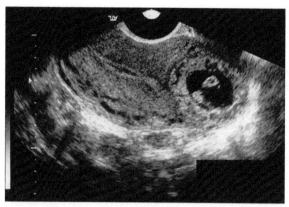

Fig. 26. Interstitial ectopic pregnancy. (*From* Advincula AP, Senapati S. Interstitial pregnancy. Fertil Steril 2004;82(6):1660–1; with permission.)

Nonviable Pregnancy

Ultrasound can detect a failed pregnancy. The most straightforward diagnosis is intrauterine fetal demise. The criteria are an embryo with a crown-rump length greater than 5 mm that has no heartbeat.[22] The size limit is intended to prevent technical or operator error from failing to detect a heartbeat early in pregnancy and incorrectly diagnosing an intrauterine fetal demise. In women with intrauterine fetal demise, the measured gestational age is often lower than the expected gestational age by last menstrual period because of a potential lag of days to weeks between the onset of nonviability and the onset of symptoms.

The other findings in failed pregnancy usually require serial testing. A completed miscarriage can appear as a nongravid uterus or have residual blood and tissue in the endometrial space. Retained products of conception have an appearance similar to that of pseudogestational sacs (**Fig. 27**). Making the distinction requires prior evidence of an IUP.

A blighted ovum is an anembryonic pregnancy and appears as an empty intrauterine sac. This is indistinguishable from an early pregnancy ultrasonographically. Serial

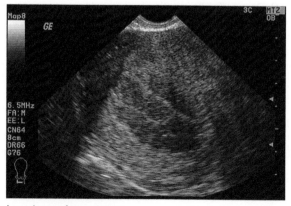

Fig. 27. Retained products of conception.

ultrasound examinations show growth of a normal gestational sac and the eventual appearance of a yolk sac and embryo, whereas a blighted ovum remains relatively unchanged unless it involutes and spontaneously aborts.

Most cases of nonviable pregnancy do not need immediate intervention, so a definitive diagnosis is rarely needed on the initial evaluation. Most cases are amenable to and require follow-up ultrasounds and serial HCG measurements to confirm a diagnosis.

Placental Abruption

Consideration must be given to the diagnosis of placental abruption in the pregnant patient who presents with the classic findings of vaginal bleeding, abdominal pain, and contractions. More subtle presentations are also seen. The patient with possible placental abruption should have a careful evaluation that includes cardiotocographic monitoring and ultrasound. Ultrasound, however, has a very low sensitivity and in itself is not able to "rule out" placental abruption. One study in women at 24 weeks or greater gestation who had sonography performed within 2 weeks of delivery found it to be 24% sensitive and 96% specific for the detection of placental abruption.[23]

SUMMARY

Bedside ultrasound has the potential to greatly improve and speed the evaluation of the symptomatic pregnant patient. Although daunting because of the variation in normal and abnormal findings, most cases are straightforward, normal IUPs. These can be imaged successfully at the novice level. The ultrasound cannot be taken in isolation. The clinical picture must also be considered. Ignoring severe pain or a history of assisted pregnancy because an IUP was present on ultrasound is to ignore the heterotopic twin.

ACKNOWLEDGMENTS

The authors thank Linda J. Kesselring, MS, ELS, for copy-editing the manuscript.

REFERENCES

1. Burgher S, Tandy T, Dawdy M. Transvaginal ultrasonography by emergency physicians decreases patient time in the emergency department. Acad Emerg Med 1998;5:802–7.
2. Lin EP, Bhatt S, Dogra VS. Diagnostic clues to ectopic pregnancy. Radiographics 2008;28:1661–71.
3. AIUM practice guideline for ultrasonography in reproductive medicine. 2008. Available at: www.aium.org/publications/guidelines/reproductiveMed.pdf. Accessed April 24, 2012.
4. Moore C, Promes SB. Ultrasound in pregnancy. Emerg Med Clin North Am 2004; 22:697–722.
5. Patel MD. "Rule out ectopic": asking the right questions, getting the right answers. Ultrasound Q 2006;22:87–100.
6. Abrams BJ, Sukumvanich P, Seibel R, et al. Ultrasound for the detection of intraperitoneal fluid: the role of Trendelenburg positioning. Am J Emerg Med 1999;17: 117–20.
7. Levine D. Ectopic pregnancy. Radiology 2007;245:385–97.
8. DeVoe RW, Pratt JH. Simultaneous intrauterine and extrauterine pregnancy. Am J Obstet Gynecol 1948;56:1119–26.

9. Bello GV, Schonholz D, Moshirpur J, et al. Combined pregnancy: the Mount Sinai experience. Obstet Gynecol Surv 1986;41:603–13.
10. Barrenetxea G, Barinaga-Rementeria L, Lopez de Larruzea A, et al. Heterotopic pregnancy: two cases and a comparative review. Fertil Steril 2007;87: 417.e9–417.e14.
11. Marcus SF, Brinsden PR. Analysis of the incidence and risk factor associated with ectopic pregnancy following in-vitro fertilization and embryo transfer. Hum Reprod 1995;10:199–203.
12. Jerrard D, Tso E, Salik R, et al. Unsuspected heterotopic pregnancy in a woman without risk factors. Am J Emerg Med 1992;10:58–60.
13. Talbot K, Simpson R, Price N, et al. Heterotopic pregnancy. J Obstet Gynaecol 2001;31:7–12.
14. Condous G, Okaro E, Khalid A, et al. The accuracy of transvaginal ultrasonography for the diagnosis of ectopic pregnancy prior to surgery. Hum Reprod 2005;20:1404–9.
15. Russell SA, Filly RA, Damato N. Sonographic diagnosis of ectopic pregnancy with endovaginal probes: what really has changed? J Ultrasound Med 1993;12: 145–51.
16. Adhikari S, Blaivas M, Lyon M. Diagnosis and management of ectopic pregnancy using bedside transvaginal ultrasonography in the ED: a 2-year experience. Am J Emerg Med 2007;25:591–6.
17. Dialani V, Levine D. Ectopic pregnancy: a review. Ultrasound Q 2004;20:105–17.
18. Blaivas M, Lyon M. Reliability of adnexal mass mobility in distinguishing possible ectopic pregnancy from corpus luteum cysts. J Ultrasound Med 2005;24: 599–603.
19. Bhatt S, Ghazale H, Dogra VS. Sonographic evaluation of ectopic pregnancy. Radiol Clin North Am 2007;45:549–60.
20. Bouyer J, Coste J, Fernandez H, et al. Sites of ectopic pregnancy: a 10 year population-based study of 1800 cases. Hum Reprod 2002;17:3224–30.
21. Ash A, Ko P, Dewar C, et al. Eccentrically located intrauterine pregnancy misdiagnosed as interstitial ectopic pregnancy. Ann Emerg Med 2010;56:684–6.
22. Albayram F, Hmaper UM. First trimester obstetric emergencies: spectrum of sonographic findings. J Clin Ultrasound 2002;30:161–77.
23. Glantz C, Purnell L. Clinical utility of sonography in the diagnosis and treatment of placental abruption. J Ultrasound Med 2002;21:837–40.

Gynecologic and Other Infections in Pregnancy

Mercedes Torres, MD*, Siamak Moayedi, MD

KEYWORDS

- Obstetrics • Infection • Antimicrobials • Vaginitis • Cervicitis • Herpes simplex virus
- Urinary tract infection • Pyelonephritis

KEY POINTS

- In obstetric patients, bacterial vaginosis and *Trichomonas vaginalis* infections should be treated only when they are symptomatic, whereas gonorrhea and chlamydial infections should be treated whenever they are detected.
- Herpes simplex virus infection should be treated and monitored closely throughout pregnancy to prevent vertical transmission.
- Regardless of the presence of symptoms, infections of the urinary tract have been associated with significant morbidity for obstetric patients and should be treated in all cases.
- Although pyelonephritis in pregnant patients traditionally requires hospital admission, a select population may be appropriate for outpatient management, provided close follow-up is available.
- Obstetric patients infected with human immunodeficiency virus on antiretroviral therapy often experience increased medication side effects such as vomiting, lactic acidosis, and hepatitis.
- All pregnant patients presenting with influenza should be treated with antivirals regardless of the timing of presentation; initiation within 48 hours after the onset of symptoms is most effective.

INTRODUCTION

Pregnant women and their fetuses are at increased risk for significant morbidity and mortality as a result of infections. Common gynecologic infections (eg, with *Neisseria gonorrhoeae*, *Chlamydia trachomatis*, herpes simplex virus [HSV], and *Trichomonas*) can cause substantial complications in pregnancy, including premature rupture of membranes, preterm delivery, and fetal malformations. Urinary tract infections (UTIs) in pregnant patients are inherently complicated and can accelerate rapidly to

Funding sources/Conflicts of interest: None.
Department of Emergency Medicine, University of Maryland School of Medicine, 110 South Paca Street, Sixth Floor, Suite 200, Baltimore, MD 21201, USA
* Corresponding author.
E-mail address: mercedet@gmail.com

pyelonephritis. Furthermore, nongynecologic infections such as those caused by the human immunodeficiency virus (HIV), influenza viruses, *Parvovirus*, and *Listeria* have serious, life-threatening implications for the fetus and mother when they occur during pregnancy. Treatment decisions for common gynecologic and nongynecologic infections must weigh the benefits of treatment against the risks of antimicrobials during pregnancy. Many of these decisions are made by emergency physicians caring for pregnant patients with acute infectious symptoms. This article highlights the most recent literature regarding the emergency department (ED) management of a variety of infections, with a focus on the pregnant patient.

INFECTIONS PRESENTING WITH VAGINAL DISCHARGE
Gonorrhea and Chlamydial Infections

Untreated gonorrhea and chlamydial infections can cause significant complications for pregnant patients, including preterm delivery, premature rupture of membranes, and perinatal mortality.[1] Data from 2010 documented the median positive test rate for chlamydia in prenatal clinics at 7.2% (range, 2.7%–21.2%), whereas the rate for gonorrhea was 0.9% (range, 0%–4.2%).[2] Gonorrhea appears to be less common, but the risks associated with it, especially during pregnancy, are more severe and include spontaneous septic abortion, chorioamnionitis, and postpartum infections. By contrast, chlamydial infection has not been shown to increase the risk of such complications.[1]

Pregnant women at increased risk of becoming infected with *N gonorrhoeae* and chlamydia are those who are single, adolescent, poor, drug abusers, or prostitutes, and those who lack prenatal care. Up to 40% of women with gonorrhea have coexisting chlamydial infection.[1] Clinical manifestations of gonorrhea and chlamydial infection in pregnant patients range from a complete lack of symptoms to cervicitis and pelvic inflammatory disease (PID).[3] Pregnant women who are asymptomatic or present with cervicitis can be treated with the outpatient regimen outlined in **Table 1**. The Centers for Disease Control and Prevention (CDC) recommends retesting for all pregnant patients with chlamydia 3 to 4 weeks following treatment to demonstrate cure. Therefore, all pregnant patients treated for chlamydia in the ED should be advised to follow up with their obstetrician for repeat testing approximately 1 month later.[3]

Pregnant patients with PID should be admitted to the hospital for administration of parenteral antibiotics. Professional societies representing obstetricians, family physicians, and infectious disease experts all recommend aggressive treatment for PID in pregnancy, dispelling the myth that PID cannot occur in pregnant women.[4] Because

Table 1 Antibiotics for chlamydial infections and gonorrhea without pelvic inflammatory disease	
Organism	**Antibiotic Recommended**
Chlamydia	Azithromycin, 1 g PO × 1 dose, or Amoxicillin, 500 mg PO TID × 7 days
Neisseria gonorrhoeae	Ceftriaxone, 250 mg IM × 1 dose, or Cefixime, 400 mg PO × 1 dose, or Azithromycin, 2 g PO × 1 dose

Abbreviations: IM, intramuscular; PO, by mouth; TID, 3 times a day.

Data from Hollier LM, Workowski K. Treatment of sexually transmitted infections in women. Infect Dis Clin North Am 2008;22:665–91; Centers for Disease Control and Prevention. Sexually transmitted diseases treatment guidelines, 2010. MMWR 2010;59(RR–12):1–116; and Biggs WS, Williams RM. Common gynecologic infections. Prim Care Clin Office Pract 2009;36:33–51.

PID is a clinical diagnosis, the CDC recommends the treatment of women who are at risk for the disease and have pelvic or lower abdominal pain, no other identifiable cause, and at least one of the following on examination: cervical motion tenderness, uterine tenderness, or adnexal tenderness.[3] The treatment of PID in pregnancy is complicated by the inability to use doxycycline. Therefore, CDC treatment regimen B is recommended to cover chlamydial infection and gonorrhea: clindamycin, 900 mg intravenously every 8 hours, and weight-based dosing of gentamicin.[3]

Bacterial Vaginosis

Bacterial vaginosis (BV) is a common cause of vaginal discharge and vaginal odor in women. BV during pregnancy is associated with an increased risk of preterm labor and delivery, premature rupture of membranes, postpartum endometritis, and chorioamnionitis. Women with a history of any of these problems are considered high-risk patients if infected with BV, regardless of their symptomatology. As a result, multiple trials have been performed to evaluate the efficacy of treating asymptomatic pregnant patients. The results of these trials have been conflicting and inconclusive. Overall, the evidence shows no benefit to treatment of asymptomatic low-risk pregnant patients who test positive for BV.[1,3,4] Some evidence suggests that treating BV in patients at high risk for preterm delivery reduces the risk of this outcome by 25% to 75%.[3] This effect has been shown primarily in women treated before 20 weeks' gestation.[1]

In symptomatic obstetric patients presenting with vaginal discharge or malodor, treatment for BV is recommended, and cure rates are estimated at approximately 70%.[1] Multiple studies have demonstrated the safety of metronidazole in pregnancy. Obstetric patients with symptomatic BV should be treated with oral metronidazole (**Table 2**). Topical therapies are not recommended for pregnant patients, because they are not as effective against infection of the upper genital tract.[3]

Trichomonas Vaginalis

It is estimated that 7% to 13% of pregnant patients are infected with *Trichomonas vaginalis*.[1] Similar to BV, *Trichomonas* infection has been associated with various morbidities in pregnant patients, including premature rupture of membranes, preterm

Table 2
Recommended treatment regimens for common causes of vaginitis

Infection Causing Vaginal Discharge	Recommended Regimen
Bacterial vaginosis	Metronidazole, 500 mg PO BID × 7 days, or Metronidazole, 250 mg PO TID × 7 days, or Clindamycin, 300 mg PO BID × 7 days
Trichomonas vaginalis	Metronidazole, 2 g PO × 1 dose, or Metronidazole, 500 mg PO BID × 7 days
Candidal vulvovaginitis	Clotrimazole, 1% cream, 5 g intravaginally × 7 days, or Miconazole, 2% cream, 5 g intravaginally × 7 days, or Terconazole, 0.4% cream, 5 g intravaginally × 7 days, or Miconazole, 100 mg vaginal suppository daily × 7 days

Abbreviation: BID, twice a day.

Data from Hollier LM, Workowski K. Treatment of sexually transmitted infections in women. Infect Dis Clin North Am 2008;22:665–91; Centers for Disease Control and Prevention. Sexually transmitted diseases treatment guidelines, 2010. MMWR 2010;59(RR–12):1–116; and Biggs WS, Williams RM. Common gynecologic infections. Prim Care Clin Office Pract 2009;36:33–51.

delivery, and low birth weight. Although the data regarding the risks of infection are clear, studies have not demonstrated a decrease in perinatal morbidity after treatment.[1] Furthermore, some evidence demonstrates an increased risk of preterm labor in women with asymptomatic infection who received treatment. Therefore, treatment is recommended for women with significant symptoms at the treating physician's discretion.[4] The metronidazole regimen outlined in **Table 2** is the recommended antimicrobial strategy, as tinidazole's safety in pregnancy is unknown.

Candidal Vulvovaginitis

Candidal vulvovaginitis is a common cause of vaginal discharge in patients presenting to urgent care clinics. Although the symptoms may be uncomfortable and distressing for patients, this condition is not associated with significant morbidity in pregnancy. Multiple topical treatment options are available for symptomatic pregnant patients. The over-the-counter and prescription topical antifungals listed in **Table 2** are all safe and effective for use in pregnancy at the indicated doses. At least 7 days of therapy are recommended for symptomatic obstetric patients to ensure adequate eradication of infection.[3]

OTHER GYNECOLOGIC INFECTIONS
Herpes Simplex Virus 1 and 2

HSV 1 and 2 can cause chronic recurrent infections in the genital region. Although HSV 2 is typically associated with genital herpes, HSV 1 has demonstrated an increasing incidence of genital involvement in recent years. One in 5 adults in the United States is infected with HSV. The overall prevalence in women is twice that of men (22% in women vs 11% among men). In the pregnant population, 22% have been shown to be infected with HSV at the beginning of their pregnancies, while 2% acquire HSV during pregnancy.[5] Pregnant women who acquire HSV during pregnancy experience more severe disease manifestations, including gingivostomatitis, vulvovaginitis, and disseminated herpes (hepatitis, encephalitis, thrombocytopenia, leukopenia, and coagulopathy). If disseminated herpes develops, the maternal mortality rate is as high as 50%.[5] Recurrent infections are more common and less severe than primary infection in pregnant women.[1,3] Recurrences typically last 7 to 10 days and more commonly occur with HSV 2.

The treatment of HSV outbreaks, whether primary or recurrent, differs during pregnancy. Acyclovir is the only antiviral with data to support its safety in pregnancy. It is typically recommended for primary, recurrent, and suppressive therapy during pregnancy (**Table 3**).[3] Famcyclovir and valacyclovir have not been evaluated adequately

Table 3
Antiviral regimens for HSV 1 and 2

Clinical Scenario	Antiviral Regimen
First outbreak of genital herpes	Acyclovir, 400 mg PO TID × 7–10 days, or Acyclovir, 200 mg PO 5 times daily × 7–10 days
Suppressive therapy for recurrent herpes	Acyclovir, 400 mg PO BID
Episodic therapy for recurrent herpes	Acyclovir, 400 mg TID × 5 days, or Acyclovir, 800 mg PO BID × 5 days, or Acyclovir, 800 mg PO TID × 2 days

Data from Centers for Disease Control and Prevention. Sexually transmitted diseases treatment guidelines, 2010. MMWR 2010;59(RR–12):1–116.

for use in pregnant patients. However, recent research has demonstrated improved bioavailability and less frequent dosing offered by valacyclovir, which may make this a more attractive option for pregnant patients once safety has been proved.[6]

The vertical transmission rates of HSV vary with the chronicity of infection. Pregnant women with primary HSV have a significantly higher risk of vertical transmission. The risk appears to be focused in the last half of pregnancy, most notably at more than 36 weeks' gestation, as the rate of transmission is 30% to 50% when there is an active primary outbreak during delivery.[1] Conversely, women who experience primary HSV infection during the first 20 weeks of their pregnancy have a vertical transmission rate of less than 1%.[1,3] Recurrent HSV infections with active lesions at the time of delivery have a vertical transmission rate of 3%, whereas those with no active lesions visualized at the time of delivery demonstrate less than 1% transmission to the newborn. Given these features, current recommendations note that all women should be evaluated for the presence of lesions or prodromal symptoms at the time of the onset of labor. If either of these exists, cesarean section delivery is recommended before the rupture of membranes or within 4 to 6 hours after rupture in women who present with ruptured membranes.[5,6]

Human Papillomavirus

Human papillomavirus (HPV) causes cervical cancer and genital warts, depending on the subtype involved. Cervical cancer is typically identified and managed in the outpatient obstetric clinic setting; pregnant women may present to the ED with genital warts. These warts often increase in size and number during pregnancy. In most cases, they are not treated during pregnancy, because the usual topical therapies are contraindicated. If the warts obscure the birth canal, trichloroacetic acid or bichloroacetic acid in 85% alcohol solution can be used to eradicate them, although this therapy is most effective for smaller lesions.[1] Most cases should be referred to an obstetrician to determine if therapy is indicated. HPV infection alone, without evidence of severe obstruction of the birth canal, is not an indication for cesarean delivery.[1]

Although there is no clear association, HPV infection has been found in the mothers of infants with recurrent respiratory papillomatosis, characterized by hoarseness and respiratory distress. HPV 6 and 11 have been associated with the development of this illness, although no clear data on vertical transmission exist.[1]

The quadrivalent HPV vaccine (active for HPV 6/11/16/18) is a Category B medication, but is not recommended for use in pregnancy. According to its manufacturers, women found to be pregnant at any point in the 3-dose immunization process should defer additional doses until after their pregnancy is complete. In a recent review of 5 phase III clinical trials of the HPV vaccine, the incidence of congenital anomalies in fetuses exposed to the vaccine in utero was not increased. Further evidence demonstrates no change in the rate of miscarriage or stillbirth among mothers who receive the HPV vaccine.[7] To date, however, the HPV vaccine is not recommended for pregnant women, owing to the lack of safety data.

Syphilis

Although adequate and definitive treatment has existed for a long time, syphilis rates have shown recent increases.[1] Therefore, the CDC continues to recommend that all women should be screened for syphilis during their first prenatal visit. In populations with poor access to prenatal care, the screening should be done at the time that pregnancy is determined, which often occurs in the ED.[3] Nontreponemal antibody tests (such as rapid plasma reagin or Venereal Disease Research Laboratory) are typically performed initially. If the result is positive, follow-up confirmatory testing with a treponemal test is recommended. Titers measured by the nontreponemal tests are proportional to disease activity.

Once diagnosed, syphilis is treated based on stage, using the same treatment guidelines as for nonpregnant patients (**Table 4**).[3] Pregnant women with primary, secondary, or early latent syphilis have an increased rate of treatment failure; therefore, a second dose of benzathine penicillin G is recommended 1 week after the first. Women with penicillin allergies should undergo desensitization and then be treated according to the guidelines. No other antibiotics are safe in pregnancy, and effective in treating maternal syphilis and preventing congenital syphilis.[1,2] If syphilis goes untreated during pregnancy, it can result in spontaneous abortion, stillbirth, fetal hydrops, intrauterine growth restriction, premature delivery, and perinatal mortality. Infants born after acquiring syphilis exhibit a wide range of problems, including hepatosplenomegaly, bone abnormalities, petechiae, anemia, jaundice, frontal bossing, palatal deformations, and nasal deformities.

The highest risk of treatment failure occurs in women who have high maternal serology titers, those who experience preterm delivery, and those who deliver shortly after receiving treatment.[1] Ultrasound imaging to look for evidence of congenital syphilis is recommended for all women diagnosed after 20 weeks of gestation. Ultrasonographic abnormalities associated with congenital syphilis include hepatomegaly, hydrops, ascites, and thickened placenta. These findings predict a greater risk of failure of fetal treatment.[3]

Bartholin Gland Cysts and Abscesses

The Bartholin glands are structures located at the 4 o'clock and 8 o'clock positions of the entrance to the vagina. When a Bartholin gland duct becomes blocked, cysts and subsequent abscess can form. Cysts are benign, uninfected collections of fluid, which are typically small and asymptomatic. In women younger than 40 years, these cysts require no intervention and respond to frequent sitz baths. For women older than 40 there is a small risk of adenocarcinoma within these cysts, so biopsy may be warranted. Infection can develop in blocked Bartholin glands, leading to abscess formation.[8]

Bartholin gland infections are typically polymicrobial and respond well to broad-spectrum antibiotics. There is no consensus regarding which antimicrobials are most effective against these infections, but polypharmacy is common. Amoxicillin-clavulanate is a reasonable option if the patient has systemic symptoms or the clinician is concerned about progression of the infection.[9] Cultures for chlamydia and *N gonorrhoeae* should be requested on drainage, but these organisms are an infrequent

Table 4	
Treatment guidelines for syphilis based on stage	
Stage of Disease	**Antibiotic Recommended**
Primary or secondary	Benzathine penicillin G, 2.4 million units IM (1 dose)
Early latent syphilis	Benzathine penicillin G, 2.4 million units IM (1 dose)
Late or unknown latent syphilis	Benzathine penicillin G, 2.4 million units IM (once weekly × 3 doses)
Neurosyphilis or ocular syphilis	Aqueous crystalline penicillin G, 18–24 million units per day, given as 3 or 4 million units IV every 4 h or continuous infusion, for 10–14 days

Abbreviation: IV, intravenous.

Data from Centers for Disease Control and Prevention. Sexually transmitted diseases treatment guidelines, 2010. MMWR 2010;59(RR–12):1–116.

cause of this infection. All of the typical interventions for Bartholin cysts and abscesses, such as incision with Word catheter placement, marsupialization, silver nitrate insertion, carbon dioxide laser therapy, and excision are safe to perform in pregnant patients. These procedures introduce an increased risk of bleeding in pregnant patients, given the increased blood flow to the pelvic region. Therefore, many providers choose to wait until after delivery, if possible, to intervene surgically. Especially in the case of a later third-trimester presentation of abscess, incision and drainage should be avoided if at all possible to decrease the risk of ascending infection that causes peripartum endometritis.[8]

Endometritis

The timeline for development of postpartum endometritis (an infection of the endometrium) ranges from a few hours to 2 weeks after delivery. Approximately 10% of cesarean deliveries and 5% of vaginal deliveries are complicated by endometritis. In contrast to other causes of postpartum fever, endometritis predictably causes a parallel increase in body temperature and heart rate. Patients present anywhere from 24 hours to several weeks postpartum with the clinical signs listed in **Box 1**.[10]

The ED workup of a postpartum woman with a clinical presentation suggestive of endometritis should include a complete blood count (CBC), comprehensive metabolic panel, coagulation studies, type and screen, catheterized urine analysis and culture (to avoid lochia contamination), and possibly computed tomography or ultrasound imaging.[10] No imaging can definitively diagnose endometritis, but imaging modalities can be useful to rule out other postpartum complications such as abscess, hematoma, and fistula. Blood cultures are not recommended in cases of endometritis, as they have not been shown to alter therapy or antibiotic choice.[11] In most cases, the emergency physician should consider and rule out the other causes of postpartum fever (**Box 2**) based on the history and physical examination.[10]

The mechanism of infection is primarily ascent of vaginal flora; therefore, antibiotic coverage for anaerobic bacterium is important. If cesarean section was performed, endometritis can be caused by coexisting skin flora and incisional infections.[10] Recommended antibiotic regimens are presented in **Table 5**. Almost all patients with suspected postpartum endometritis should be admitted for administration of parenteral antibiotics, unless they exhibit very mild clinical symptoms and are several weeks past their delivery.[10]

Box 1
Clinical signs of postpartum endometritis

- Temperature higher than 101°F (38.3°C)
- Temperature higher than 100.4°F (38°C) on 2 occasions at least 6 hours apart
- Tachycardia paralleling the increase in body temperature
- Uterine tenderness
- Midline lower abdominal pain
- Purulent lochia
- Headache
- Malaise
- Anorexia

Data from Faro S. Postpartum endometritis. Clin Perinatol 2005;32:803–14.

Box 2
Causes of postpartum fever

- Surgical-site infection (episiotomy, laceration, or cesarean section incision)
- Deep vein thrombosis/pulmonary embolism
- Pyelonephritis
- Mastitis
- Colitis due to *Clostridium difficile* infection
- Drug fever
- Viral illness

Septic Abortion

After spontaneous or elective abortions, women are at risk for uterine infection related to retained products of conception or nonsterile technique. These patients frequently present to the ED with fever, tachycardia, uterine tenderness, foul-smelling vaginal discharge or vaginal bleeding, and abdominal pain. The history often reveals a recent termination of pregnancy or complications leading to miscarriage. The mechanism for this infection, similar to postpartum endometritis, is ascent of vaginal flora into the uterine cavity through an open cervical os.[12]

In addition to blood work and urine and cervical cultures, ultrasound imaging is the diagnostic modality of choice for detecting retained products of conception or retained foreign bodies. Intravenous administration of antibiotics is recommended in the ED while the patient is being prepared for a dilation and curettage (D&C) procedure to remove any retained contents and eradicate the source of endotoxin contributing to the infection. In this case, coverage for gram-positive, gram-negative, and anaerobic bacteria is recommended. Typical regimens include a penicillin or cephalosporin for gram-positive coverage, coupled with an aminoglycoside for gram-negative organisms, and clindamycin or metronidazole for anaerobic coverage. From the ED, these patients typically go to the operating room for the D&C and are subsequently admitted for intravenous antimicrobial therapy.[12]

INFECTIONS OF THE URINARY TRACT
Asymptomatic Bacteriuria

Asymptomatic bacteriuria (ASB) occurs in 2% to 10% of pregnant women. If left untreated, pyelonephritis will develop in 15% to 45% of these women, which causes

---

Table 5
Initial antibiotic regimens for the treatment of postpartum endometritis

Route of Administration	Antibiotics Recommended
Intravenous (breastfeeding)	Clindamycin, 900 mg every 8 h, and Gentamicin, 5 mg/kg every 24 h, and Ampicillin, 2 g every 6 h
Intravenous (not breastfeeding)	Gentamicin, 5 mg/kg every 24 h, and Ampicillin, 2 g every 6 h, and Metronidazole, 500 mg every 8 h
Oral	Amoxicillin-clavulanate, 875 mg PO BID × 7 days

Data from Faro S. Postpartum endometritis. Clin Perinatol 2005;32:803–14.

significant maternal and neonatal morbidities. The most common pathogen found on urine culture for pregnant women with ASB is *Escherichia coli*. Others include *Staphylococcus saprophyticus*, *Klebsiella* spp, *Enterobacter* spp, *Proteus* spp, and *Enterococcus* spp.[13]

The recommended method of obtaining 2 consecutive positive urine cultures demonstrating the same organism with greater than 100,000 colony-forming units per milliliter of urine is impractical for emergency practice. As a result, other diagnostic modalities have been adopted for this purpose. The widely available and relatively simple urine dipstick test has been evaluated as a more practical method for detecting ASB in pregnant patients in the ED. Although conflicting data exist regarding its reliability, a positive nitrite test has a high level of accuracy for identifying patients with ASB. Concurrently negative nitrites and leukocyte esterase tests can effectively rule out ASB in pregnant patients.[14] The dipslide is a rapid culture test that can be performed in an outpatient setting. The results specify colony counts of gram-negative bacteria on the surface of a slide dipped into a urine specimen. A positive test indicates a high likelihood of ASB whereas a negative test rules it out.[14]

Treatment of ASB in pregnant patients decreases the incidence of pyelonephritis and low birth weight.[15] Given the evolving resistance to antimicrobials previously effective for infections of the urinary tract, knowledge of local resistance patterns is helpful in determining the antibiotic of choice, especially in the ED, where culture results are often unavailable. Ampicillin and sulfonamides are not recommended because of the high prevalence of resistant *E coli* strains. Nitrofurantoin, cephalosporins, and fosfomycin have proved to be effective and safe in most circumstances.[14] Although some reports suggest no increase in treatment failures with a 1-day regimen, a recent Cochrane review and guidelines from the Infectious Diseases Society of America recommend a 3- to 7-day course of antibiotics when possible until more definitive research determines the efficacy of the 1-day regimen.[13,16]

Symptomatic Urinary Tract Infections and Pyelonephritis

UTIs are one of the most common infectious problems during pregnancy, affecting 20% of all pregnant women.[17] Pyelonephritis is the most common indication for hospitalization of pregnant women.[18] The infecting pathogens are the same as those found in most cases of ASB. *E coli* has been implicated in approximately 70% to 85% of cases, followed by *Klebsiella* spp, *Enterobacter* spp, *Proteus* spp, *Enterococcus faecalis*, and group B streptococci.

Women at increased risk for developing pyelonephritis in pregnancy include those with neurogenic bladder, incompetent vesiculoureteral valves, diabetes mellitus, or sickle cell disease. In addition, significant physiologic changes that occur during pregnancy contribute to the increased likelihood of developing pyelonephritis (**Box 3**).[18] Many of these changes result in stasis of urine in the ureters or bladder, creating an environment conducive to infection. Most cases of pyelonephritis occur in the second or third trimester, when these physiologic changes are most prominent.[18]

The ED evaluation of a pregnant patient with pyelonephritis should include laboratory tests to assess for renal insufficiency, anemia, and bacteremia. Any patient who is febrile (temperature >39°C), septic, or displaying symptoms of acute respiratory distress syndrome (ARDS) should have blood cultures performed. Gram-negative bacteremia can produce toxins that cause clinical deterioration in the form of ARDS, septic shock, and disseminated intravascular coagulation.[18] Additional complications of pyelonephritis during pregnancy include recurrent infections, preterm labor, premature rupture of membranes, chorioamnionitis, and neonatal fever/infection.[17]

Box 3
Physiologic changes of pregnancy that increase the risk of pyelonephritis

- Ureteral and renal calyceal dilatation due to increased progesterone level
- Ureteral compression from growth of the uterus
- Incomplete bladder emptying
- Elevations in urinary glucose
- Increased alkalization of the urine

Data from Jolley JA, Wing DA. Pyelonephritis in pregnancy: an update on treatment options for optimal outcomes. Drugs 2010;70(13):1643–55.

When evaluating a pregnant patient with pyelonephritis, identifying the best antibiotic and deciding the patient's disposition present challenges. Penicillins and cephalosporins are recommended to treat pyelonephritis in pregnant patients. Tetracyclines and fluoroquinolones are not recommended because of their side-effect profile for the fetus; however, aminoglycosides such as gentamicin are still used in severe cases. Historically, patients were hospitalized for intravenous administration of fluids and antibiotics until they were afebrile for at least 48 hours. Subsequently, they were placed on 2 weeks of oral antibiotics and had repeat urine cultures after the antibiotic regimen was complete to prove resolution of bacteriuria.[18]

More recently, ambulatory management has been used for pregnant patients with pyelonephritis. Research has demonstrated that, at less than 24 weeks' gestation, this group can be managed as outpatients (5% failure rate).[18] Conversely, 30% of patients at more than 24 weeks' gestation failed outpatient management. Further investigation revealed that a select population does not require admission and can be treated as outpatients for pyelonephritis during pregnancy (**Box 4**). Patients who meet these criteria are typically managed during a period of observation in the ED initially, with intravenous hydration, intravenous or intramuscular administration of antibiotics, and laboratory work. If the CBC and basic metabolic panel (BMP) are normal and the patient can tolerate an oral challenge, she can be discharged to follow-up with her obstetrician/gynecologist or asked to return to the ED in 24 hours for an additional intramuscular dose of antibiotics (usually ceftriaxone).[18] At the 24-hour follow-up visit, if the patient appears to be well and improving, the physician can begin oral antibiotics for a total of 10 days. After completion of the antibiotic course, a urine culture should be obtained to demonstrate resolution of the bacteriuria. In addition, antibiotic prophylaxis against recurrence is recommended. Nitrofurantoin (100 mg by mouth PO every afternoon) or cephalexin (250–500 mg by mouth every afternoon) is recommended for this purpose and should be continued until 4 to

---

Box 4
Patients eligible for outpatient management of pyelonephritis

- Less than 24 weeks' gestation
- Otherwise healthy
- Without fever, nausea, vomiting, tachycardia, tachypnea, or hypotension

Data from Jolley JA, Wing DA. Pyelonephritis in pregnancy: an update on treatment options for optimal outcomes. Drugs 2010;70(13):1643–55.

6 weeks postpartum. Monthly urine cultures are also suggested as a surveillance technique.[18]

OTHER CLINICALLY IMPORTANT INFECTIONS IN PREGNANCY
Human Immunodeficiency Virus and Antiretroviral Therapy

The management of HIV during pregnancy is a complicated clinical scenario involving the input of obstetricians and infectious disease specialists. Emergency physicians can become involved when patients present with acute issues related to antiretroviral (ARV) therapy. Such issues include a new diagnosis of pregnancy in an HIV-infected woman, managing first trimester nausea and vomiting in patients on ARV therapy, recognizing and treating ARV toxicities, and managing precipitous labor in an HIV-infected mother.[19,20]

Although it is recommended that all HIV-infected pregnant women receive ARV therapy during pregnancy, the ED is not the appropriate setting for its initiation. When an emergency physician identifies pregnancy in an HIV-infected woman, the most appropriate course of action is to ensure rapid follow-up with an obstetrician and an infectious disease specialist. For women presenting before 14 weeks' gestation with well-managed HIV infection and not on ARV therapy, there is time to schedule these outpatient appointments. These patients should not start ARV therapy until after 14 weeks to decrease the risk of teratogenicity and allow time for the nausea and vomiting that often complicate the first trimester to subside. However, if a pregnancy of more than 14 weeks is detected in an HIV-infected patient who is on ARV therapy, or who requires initiation of ARV therapy for maternal health, obstetric as well as infectious disease specialist consultation is imperative. In all cases, HIV-infected women at more than 28 weeks' gestation should be on ARV therapy, regardless of their CD4 count or viral load.[19,20] The data associating ARV therapy with preterm labor and birth defects are insufficient and conflicting; therefore, the benefits of their use at this point outweigh the undetermined risks.[20]

Given the recommended universal use of ARV therapy in the second and third trimesters, care of these HIV-infected pregnant patients focuses on the management of medication toxicities and side effects. The toxic side effects of ARV therapy that pose the highest risk during pregnancy and cause the most concern are lactic acidosis, drug-induced hepatitis, and hepatic steatosis. The physiologic changes that occur during pregnancy increase the risk of these toxicities, although rates are still low overall. More specifically, pregnancy increases the risk of mitochondrial dysfunction causing acute fatty liver, HELLP syndrome (hemolysis/elevated liver enzymes/low platelet count), and lactic acidosis associated with the use of nucleoside reverse transcriptase inhibitors. Less severe side effects, which occur more commonly, include nausea, vomiting, glucose intolerance, and anemia.[20]

Laboratory studies, such as a CBC, BMP, liver function tests, and measurement of lactate level, can assist in the diagnosis and management of these toxicities. If a patient presents with severe toxicity or intractable nausea and vomiting and the decision is made to stop the ARV therapy, all ARV medications should be stopped concurrently and reinitiated at a later date by an infectious disease specialist in an attempt to avoid the development of viral resistance.[20]

If an HIV-infected patient presents to the ED in active labor, she should receive intravenous zidovudine regardless of her ARV regimen as soon as possible, before delivery. In addition, to decrease vertical transmission risks, instrumentation with fetal scalp electrodes, fetal scalp pH blood sampling, and artificial rupture of membranes should be avoided. Ideally, HIV-infected pregnant women with a viral load greater than 1000 copies/mL should have an elective prelabor cesarean section at 38 weeks' gestation.[20,21]

Methicillin-Resistant Staphylococcus aureus Infection

With the increasing prevalence of community-associated methicillin-resistant *Staphylococcus aureus* infection (MRSA), emergency physicians are faced with the challenge of managing this infection in special populations, including pregnant patients. Recent data suggest overall lower rates of MRSA colonization in pregnant patients (4%) than in the general population (20%–30%). However, case series have demonstrated that MRSA is commonly isolated from vulvar abscesses and is increasing in frequency in breast infections, such as mastitis and abscess.[22] The risk of vertical transmission from MRSA-colonized mothers is very low; genital colonization has not been associated with an increase in early-onset neonatal MRSA infection.[23]

Treatment of MRSA in pregnant patients is focused on incision and drainage as well as antibiotic therapy. As in the nonobstetric population, abscesses are best managed with drainage of the cavity coupled with the prescription of antibiotics based on the size of the abscess, the extent of infection, and the patient's comorbidities. The physiologic changes of pregnancy related to the renal, gastrointestinal, hepatic, and hematologic systems all contribute to alter medication levels in the bloodstream, which can have a significant impact on antimicrobial resistance patterns. Therefore, pregnant patients should be monitored closely for their response to antimicrobial therapy, and increased doses may be preferred. The antimicrobials that are active against most strains of MRSA and safe in pregnancy include trimethoprim-sulfamethoxazole (US Food and Drug Administration category C), vancomycin (intravenous use only), clindamycin (inducible resistance is possible), and gentamicin.[22]

Influenza

Pregnant patients and those within 2 weeks postpartum are at increased risk for serious morbidity and mortality from the influenza virus. This phenomenon was demonstrated during the 2009 outbreak of H1N1 influenza, when pregnant/peripartum women were 4 times more likely than the general public to be hospitalized.[24] Data from the outbreak demonstrate that most pregnant women hospitalized with H1N1 were in their second or third trimester, and 1 in 5 required intensive care at some point in their hospitalization. In addition, although most pregnant women presenting to a provider with H1N1 initially had mild symptoms, they experienced more rapid and severe clinical deterioration than the general public. Respiratory complications, such as pneumonia and ARDS, were most prevalent among pregnant patients.[24] There is no clear evidence regarding the risk of vertical transmission of influenza, but the increased risks of preterm delivery and fetal morbidity have been demonstrated.[24,25]

Rapid influenza tests are notoriously insensitive and should not be used to determine the need for therapy, especially in high-risk populations such as pregnant women. Although the general recommendations are to initiate antiviral therapy in patients presenting within 48 hours after symptoms onset or with severe disease, all pregnant patients, regardless of the duration of their symptoms, should be offered antiviral therapy because of the increased risk of serious sequelae. Although antivirals against influenza are category C medications, their risks to the fetus are outweighed by the potential risk of influenza itself. The CDC recommends oseltamivir and zanamivir for antiviral therapy (**Table 6**). In addition, chemoprophylaxis is recommended for patients with close contact exposures, using the same 2 antivirals with slightly different dosing regimens (see **Table 6**).[25,26] Influenza vaccination by injection is the most effective strategy for decreasing the burden of this disease among pregnant

Table 6	
Antiviral therapy and chemoprophylaxis for influenza	
Indication	Antivirals Recommended
Influenza treatment	Oseltamivir, 75 mg PO BID × 5 days, or Zanamivir, 10 mg inhaled BID × 5 days
Chemoprophylaxis	Oseltamivir, 75 mg PO daily × 10 days, or Zanamivir, 10 mg inhaled daily × 10 days

Data from Centers for Disease Control and Prevention. Updated recommendations for obstetric health care providers related to use of antiviral medications in the treatment and prevention of influenza for the 2010-2011 season. In: Seasonal Influenza (Flu), December 29, 2010. Available at: www.cdc.gov/flu/professionals/antivirals/avrec_ob2011.htm. Accessed July 16, 2012.

populations, and should be emphasized during the months of high seasonal influenza activity (October to April).[24]

Parvovirus B19

Parvovirus B19 is an important infection to consider when caring for pregnant patients presenting to the ED with rash, arthralgia, and fever, given the potentially catastrophic risks to the fetus. Parvovirus B19 infection is asymptomatic in most patients. It can be characterized by the "slapped cheek" facial rash known as erythema infectiosum, a maculopapular rash on the trunk and extremities, headache, fever, and peripheral polyarthropathy of the hands, wrists, and knees. More than half of pregnant women in the United States have evidence of previous exposure to this virus, but the incidence of new infection during pregnancy ranges from 1% in nonepidemic years to 10% in epidemic years. Epidemics typically occur in a cyclic manner every 3 to 6 years.[27]

Transmission is through respiratory droplets or blood products. Vertical transmission does occur across the placenta. The highest risk of fetal demise or anemia (hydrops) appears to be early in pregnancy. When caring for a pregnant woman who may be infected acutely with parvovirus B19, it is important to request immunologic testing to determine her immune status. Women whose blood tests are positive for immunoglobulin G and negative for immunoglobulin M (IgM) antibodies demonstrate previous immunity and therefore no risk to the fetus. Positive IgM antibodies indicate acute infection. All women with positive IgM antibodies should be counseled regarding the risk of fetal anemia and death as a result of the infection.[28]

There are no effective antivirals to prevent vertical transmission or treat infection. Therefore, infected pregnant women should be referred for close follow-up with their obstetrician if the diagnosis is made or suspected in the ED. Women who are more than 20 weeks pregnant should have periodic screening ultrasound examinations for several weeks after infection to look for signs of fetal anemia. Fetal transfusion should be pursued in conjunction with maternal/fetal medicine specialists if signs of fetal anemia develop, because it can prevent significant fetal morbidity and mortality.[28]

Listeriosis

Listeriosis is primarily a food-borne illness, with outbreaks occurring most commonly during the summer months. It affects pregnant women 20 times more often than the general population. Listeriosis causes very mild symptoms for mothers, such as low-grade fever, back pain, and flu-like illness, but it can be devastating to the fetus. The case fatality rate for fetuses of infected mothers is 20% to 30%. The diagnosis of listeriosis is difficult, but critical. For any pregnant woman presenting to the ED with fever and flu-like symptoms, but without a clear diagnosis, blood cultures for *Listeria* should be considered.[29]

Emergency physicians may choose to initiate empiric therapy if they have a high clinical suspicion for this infection (such as the patient's report of recent ingestion of contaminated food). Intravenous ampicillin, in doses greater than 6 g per day, is first-line therapy. Higher doses are used to achieve adequate penetration of the placenta as well as umbilical cord, where *Listeria* can remain subsequent to treatment. In patients with true penicillin allergies, intravenous erythromycin is second-line therapy, at doses of 4 g per day. The recommended duration of therapy varies, but a minimum of 14 days has been suggested in women with listeriosis whose fetuses survive the initial insult of infection. Therefore, all pregnant patients with a high suspicion for listeriosis should have blood cultures and be admitted for intravenous administration of antibiotics until culture results return.[29]

SUMMARY

Pregnant patients are at risk for a wide range of infections that can be dangerous to their health as well as the health of the fetus. Although treatment is recommended for most of these infections, the risks of therapy to the fetus need to be weighed against the risk of untreated infection. When managing obstetric patients presenting with gynecologic infections such as those caused by *Chlamydia*, *N gonorrhoeae*, *Treponema pallidum*, and HSV, treatment is recommended even in the absence of symptoms. Obstetric patients presenting with bacteriuria, even those who are asymptomatic, should be treated with antimicrobials, given the high incidence of subsequent pyelonephritis. Similarly, infections from HIV, influenza virus, parvovirus B19, and *Listeria* should always be treated and monitored closely in pregnant patients because of the significant risks of infection to the mother and fetus. Postpartum complications such as endometritis and septic abortion require immediate parenteral therapy to prevent sepsis, disseminated intravascular coagulation, ARDS, and other life-threatening sequelae.

Other common infections in pregnancy are often not treated because the risks of treatment outweigh the benefits. For example, BV and trichomoniasis in asymptomatic pregnant patients should not be treated. The benefits of treatment for HPV and Bartholin gland infections during pregnancy are not substantial in most cases; therefore, treatment is usually deferred until the postpartum period.

REFERENCES

1. Hollier LM, Workowski K. Treatment of sexually transmitted infections in women. Infect Dis Clin North Am 2008;22:665–91.
2. Centers for disease control and prevention. STDs in women and infants. In: 2010 sexually transmitted disease surveillance. 2010. Available at: www.cdc.gov/std/stats10/womenandinf.htm#preg. Accessed July 16, 2012.
3. Centers for Disease Control, Prevention. Sexually transmitted diseases treatment guidelines, 2010. MMWR Recomm Rep 2010;59(RR–12):1–116.
4. Biggs WS, Williams RM. Common gynecologic infections. Prim Care 2009;36: 33–51.
5. Anzivino E, Fioriti D, Mischitelli M, et al. Herpes simplex virus infection in pregnancy and in neonate: status of art of epidemiology, diagnosis, therapy and prevention. Virol J 2009;6:40.

6. Roberts S. Herpes simplex virus: incidence of neonatal herpes simplex virus, maternal screening, management during pregnancy, and HIV. Curr Opin Obstet Gynecol 2009;21:124–30.
7. Garland SM, Ault KA, Gall SA, et al. Pregnancy and infant outcomes in the clinical trials of a human papilloma virus type 6/11/16/18 vaccine: a combined analysis of five randomized controlled trials. Obstet Gynecol 2009;114:1179.
8. Hill DA, Lense JJ. Office management of Bartholin gland cysts and abscesses. Am Fam Physician 1998;57(7):1611–6.
9. Bhide A, Nama V, Patel S, et al. Microbiology of cysts/abscesses of the Bartholins gland: review of empirical antibiotic therapy against microbial culture. J Obstet Gynaecol 2010;30(7):701–3.
10. Faro S. Postpartum endometritis. Clin Perinatol 2005;32:803–14.
11. Locksmith GJ, Duff P. Assessment of the value of routine blood cultures in the evaluation and treatment of patients with chorioamnionitis. Infect Dis Obstet Gynecol 1994;2:111–4.
12. Gorgas DL. Infections related to pregnancy. Emerg Med Clin North Am 2008;26: 345–66.
13. Widmer M, Gulmezoglu AM, Mignini L, et al. Duration of treatment for asymptomatic bacteriuria during pregnancy. Cochrane Database Syst Rev 2011;(12):CD000491.
14. Lumbiganon P, Laopaiboon M, Thinkhamrop J. Screening and treating asymptomatic bacteriuria in pregnancy. Curr Opin Obstet Gynecol 2010;22:95–9.
15. Smaill F, Vasquez JC. Antibiotics for asymptomatic bacteriuria in pregnancy. Cochrane Database Syst Rev 2007;(2):CD000490.
16. Nicolle LE, Bradley S, Colgan R, et al. Infectious Diseases Society of America guidelines for the diagnosis and treatment of asymptomatic bacteriuria in adults. Clin Infect Dis 2005;40:643–54.
17. Vazquez JC, Abalos E. Treatments for symptomatic urinary tract infections during pregnancy. Cochrane Database Syst Rev 2011;(1):CD002256.
18. Jolley JA, Wing DA. Pyelonephritis in pregnancy. Drugs 2010;709130:1643–55.
19. Vogler MA, Singh H, Wright R. Complex decisions in managing HIV infection during pregnancy. Curr HIV/AIDS Rep 2011;8:122–31.
20. Mirochnick M, Best BM, Clarke DF. Antiretroviral pharmacology: special issues regarding pregnant women and neonates. Clin Perinatol 2010;37:907–27.
21. Waldura JF. Prevention of perinatal HIV transmission: the Perinatal HIV Hotline perspective. Top Antivir Med 2011;19(1):23–6.
22. Beigi RH. Clinical implications of methicillin-resistant *Staphylococcus aureus* in pregnancy. Curr Opin Obstet Gynecol 2011;23:82–6.
23. Andrews WW, Schellonka R, Waites K, et al. Genital tract methicillin-resistant Staphylococcus aureus, risk of vertical transmission in pregnant women. Obstet Gynecol 2008;111:113–8.
24. Panda B, Panda A, Riley LE. Selected viral infections in pregnancy. Obstet Gynecol Clin North Am 2010;37:321–31.
25. Mosby LG, Rasmussen SA, Jamieson DJ. 2009 pandemic influenza A (H1N1) in pregnancy: a systematic review of the literature. Am J Obstet Gynecol 2011;205: 10–8.
26. Centers for Disease Control and Prevention. Updated recommendations for obstetric health care providers related to use of antiviral medications in the treatment and prevention of influenza for the 2010-2011 season. In: Seasonal Influenza (Flu), December 29, 2010. Available at: www.cdc.gov/flu/professionals/antivirals/avrec_ob2011.htm. Accessed July 16, 2012.

27. Lamont RF, Sobel JD, Vaisbuch E, et al. Parvovirus B19 infection in human pregnancy. BJOG 2011;188:175–86.

28. deJong EP, Walther FJ, Kroes AC, et al. Parvovirus B19 infection in pregnancy: new insights and management. Prenat Diagn 2011;31:419–25.

29. Janakiraman V. Listeriosis in pregnancy: diagnosis, treatment and prevention. Rev Obstet Gynecol 2008;1(4):179–85.

Nonobstetric Abdominal Pain and Surgical Emergencies in Pregnancy

Laura Diegelmann, MD, RDMS

KEYWORDS

- Acute abdominal pain • Pregnancy • Pyelonephritis • Appendicitis • Cholecystitis
- Pancreatitis • Adnexal torsion • Bowel obstruction

KEY POINTS

- Pregnant patients present a diagnostic challenge to emergency physicians.
- Physiologic changes during pregnancy can alter presentations of common pathology.
- Imaging should not be delayed when a surgical cause of abdominal pain is suspected.
- If possible, start with imaging that poses the least risk to the mother and fetus—MRI and ultrasound.

INTRODUCTION

The evaluation, work-up, and management of pregnant patients are essential in the practice of emergency medicine. Patients present to emergency departments (EDs) at different stages of pregnancy and with a variety of complaints. ED physicians must be cognizant of atypical presentations of nonobstetric causes of abdominal pain and surgical emergencies in pregnant patients. Acute abdomen develops during 1 in 500 to 635 pregnancies.[1] During pregnancy, 0.2% to 1.0% of women require general surgery for a nonobstetric problem.[2]

Several anatomic changes that occur during pregnancy cause atypical presentations. These changes, combined with a hesitancy to perform radiographic tests, create difficulties in emergency physicians' evaluations of pregnant patients. Acute abdominal pain can arise from several systems: gastrointestinal, urogenital, gynecologic, or obstetric (**Fig. 1**). Delay in diagnosis or treatment can cause harm to mother and fetus. Gastrointestinal disorders account for 0.5% to 1% of presentations requiring surgery during pregnancy.[3] In comparison, only 0.01% of pregnant women with adnexal masses require surgery to correct torsion.[4]

The author has no financial relationships that constitute or suggest a conflict of interest.
Department of Emergency Medicine, University of Maryland School of Medicine, 110 South Paca Street, 6th Floor, Suite 200, Baltimore, MD 21201, USA
E-mail address: laurad98@hotmail.com

Emerg Med Clin N Am 30 (2012) 885–901
http://dx.doi.org/10.1016/j.emc.2012.08.012
0733-8627/12/$ – see front matter © 2012 Elsevier Inc. All rights reserved.

emed.theclinics.com

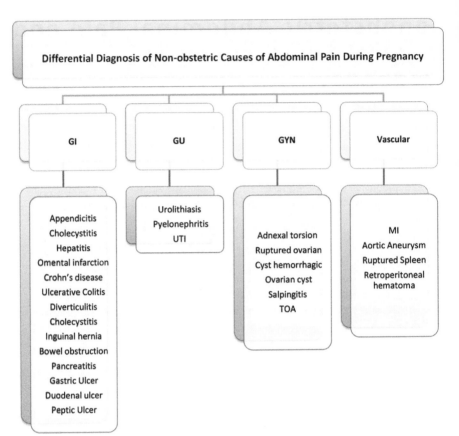

Fig. 1. Differential diagnosis of abdominal pain during pregnancy. GI, gastrointestinal; GU, genitourinary; GYN, gynecologic; MI, myocardial infarction; TOA, tubo-ovarian abscess; UTI, urinary tract infection.

ANATOMIC AND PHYSIOLOGIC CHANGES IN PREGNANCY

Pregnancy causes many changes that affect the presentation of acute abdominal pain. Heartburn and constipation are frequent complaints during pregnancy, because of decreased gastric motility. The gravid uterus, considered an abdominal organ at approximately 12 weeks' gestational age, compresses and displaces the underlying and surrounding viscera.[4] The expanding uterus makes it difficult to localize pain and can mask or delay the emergence of peritoneal signs.[2] Increased laxity of the anterior abdominal wall can also further delay peritoneal signs during pregnancy.

Progesterone prepares the body for pregnancy by relaxing smooth muscles, which is particularly important in the expanding uterus but also affects the gastrointestinal tract (**Box 1**). Progesterone relaxes the lower esophageal sphincter and decreases gastric motility, which increase the frequency of heartburn, gastroesophageal reflux, and nausea during pregnancy. The slowing of gastric motility also leads to constipation, with resultant abdominal pain. Progesterone has the same slowing effect on the gallbladder, causing stasis of the bile and increasing the incidence of cholelithiasis and resultant cholecystitis. Additionally, elevated levels of estrogen increase the concentration of bile, which also increases the formation of cholelithiasis and risk of acute cholecystitis.[1]

Box 1
Effects of progesterone during pregnancy
• Lowers esophageal sphincter relaxation
◦ Heartburn
◦ Nausea
◦ Reflux
• Decreases gastric motility
◦ Constipation
• Causes gallbladder stasis
◦ Sludging of bile
◦ Cholelithiasis
◦ Cholecystitis

PATHOPHYSIOLOGY
Pyelonephritis

A urinary tract infection (UTI) is an infection anywhere along the urinary tract, affecting the bladder, ureter, or kidneys. A UTI is most often caused by a bacterial pathogen and presents as a combination of symptoms: urinary frequency, urgency, or burning. Asymptomatic bacteriuria, that is, the presence of bacteria in a clean-catch urine sample without the typical symptoms or signs of a UTI, is the most common UTI in pregnant women.[5] The Infectious Diseases Society of America established 2 criteria as components of asymptomatic bacteriuria[6]:

- Two consecutive voided urine specimens in which the same bacteria are isolated in quantitative counts of $\geq 10^5$ CFU/mL (in women)
- A single catheterized urine specimen with one bacterial species isolated in a quantitative count of $\geq 10^2$ CFU/mL (in women and men)

Although pregnancy itself does not increase the presence of bacteria in urine, the changes that occur during pregnancy increase the risk of complications from bacteriuria. Pregnant women are especially likely to develop pyelonephritis, an infection of the upper urinary tract.[5] The diagnosis of acute pyelonephritis (APN) is based on a combination of the following clinical symptoms and laboratory data:

- Fever (temperature $\geq 38°C$)
- Flank pain
- Costovertebral angle tenderness
- Bacteriuria or pyuria revealed by urinalysis

Pyuria is indicated by an increased number of polymorphonuclear leukocytes in the urine, suggesting an inflammatory response of the urinary tract.[6] APN is most often caused by *Escherichia coli* and found in pregnant women who are young, nulliparous, and in their second trimester.[7,8]

The Infectious Diseases Society of America recommends the following guidelines for evaluating pregnant women for pyelonephritis[6]:

- Pregnant women should be screened for bacteriuria by urine culture at least once in the early stages of pregnancy; if the results are positive, they should be treated with an antibiotic.

- The duration of antimicrobial therapy (nitrofurantoin or a sulfonamide) should be 3 to 7 days.
- After treatment, periodic screening for recurrent bacteriuria should be performed.
- No recommendation can be made for or against repeated screening of culture-negative women. in the later stages of pregnancy.

Pregnant women are susceptible to APN because of ureteral dilation that begins in the early stages of pregnancy and persists until the postpartum period. There are 2 proposed mechanisms for this increased risk. The first is that the increased levels of progesterone relax the smooth muscles of the ureters, causing dilation. The second mechanism is from compression of the ureters by the enlarging uterus, causing dilation. This dilation is less pronounced on the left because of the protection from the overlying colon. Slowed peristalsis and dilation of the ureter lead to urinary stasis, which increases not only the risk of infection but also the incidence of kidney stone formation.[4]

Imaging is usually not indicated in uncomplicated pyelonephritis and is reserved for patients who do not respond to antibiotics or who have recurrent or severe symptoms. If imaging confirms the diagnosis or reveals complications of APN, then CT, ultrasound, and radiography with intravenous urography can be used. In pregnant women, it is best to limit radiation exposure; therefore, ultrasound is preferred as the initial imaging modality. The kidney often appears normal on ultrasound, but certain subtle findings can be detected.[9] In the standard 2-D mode, findings consistent with APN include the following:

- Variation in the echogenicity of the parenchyma (usually hyperechoic)
- Loss of corticomedullary differentiation
- Decrease in visualization of renal sinus fat
- Urothelial thickening
- Intraparenchymal gas

The color and power Doppler modes allow detection of decreased perfusion in the affected parenchyma. While scanning the kidney with ultrasound, it is especially important to look for the complications of APN: intrarenal or perinephric abscess, calculi, and obstruction, as suggested by the presence of hydronephrosis (**Fig. 2**).

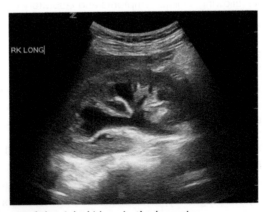

Fig. 2. Hydronephrosis of the right kidney in the long view.

Appendicitis

Appendicitis is one of the most common problems in pregnant women with acute abdomen. Appendicitis occurs in approximately 1 of every 1500 pregnancies.[2,4] The women in whom acute appendicitis develops during pregnancy most commonly present in the second trimester.[10,11] Pregnancy does not confer a greater risk of developing appendicitis, because the incidence of appendicitis is the same in pregnant and nonpregnant women.[12,13] Pregnancy is associated, however, with an increased rate of rupture of the appendix, which occurs 2 or 3 times more frequently than in nonpregnant women.[14] A perforated appendix increases fetal morbidity and mortality rates, which are as high as 20% to 35% with perforation and as low as 0% to 1.5% in uncomplicated appendicitis.[15]

Unlike other causes of abdominal pain in pregnancy (eg, cholecystitis, pyelonephritis, and intestinal obstruction), appendicitis is always a surgical emergency. Pregnancy complicates the diagnosis of appendicitis because its false-negative rate can be as high as 55% among pregnant women compared with the 10% to 30% rate found among nonpregnant women.[11]

Physiologic changes during pregnancy further complicate the diagnosis. Many women present with nausea, vomiting, and anorexia, which are not uncommon symptoms during pregnancy. A relative increase in blood volume can delay the development of tachycardia and hypotension during an acutely worsening or rupturing appendicitis. Laboratory tests might show leukocytosis, a common physiologic change during pregnancy,[16] but an astute emergency physician should not depend on fever and leukocytosis for the diagnosis of acute appendicitis.[10,17] The appendix might move during pregnancy, causing pain to be experienced in an atypical location.[11] Most studies agree, however, that, overall, the most common complaint during pregnancy in women later confirmed to have appendicitis is right lower quadrant pain.[17-19]

Diagnosing appendicitis during pregnancy causes another dilemma: the clinician must weigh the risk of rupture from a delay in diagnosis versus the risk of exposing the fetus to radiation. CT is the gold standard for diagnosing appendicitis in nonpregnant patients, but it is often avoided during pregnancy.[20] As ultrasound becomes an increasingly available diagnostic tool in EDs, it is used more often to diagnose conditions, such as appendicitis. Ultrasound does have limitations, however, such as body habitus, intraluminal air, and operator level of experience.[20] The use of ultrasound for appendicitis involves graded compression along the cecum to evaluate the compressibility of the appendix.[21,22] This technique is less useful after week 35 of pregnancy because of the technical difficulties of compressing the appendix.[23] In addition, the gravid uterus often alters abdominal contents, distorting common anatomy and landmarks for the ultrasonographer.[24] Several studies have shown that additional work-up is not needed when ultrasound is positive for appendicitis.[10,22] But if ultrasound is negative or nondiagnostic, then additional work-up with MRI or CT or further observation is warranted (**Figs. 3** and **4**). Several investigators have recommended MRI as either the initial diagnostic tool or the imaging choice after a nondiagnostic or negative ultrasound scan.[20,24-27] Ultimately, clinical suspicion, physician impression, and physical and diagnostic examinations should aid in the diagnosis of acute appendicitis, and surgical consultation should not be delayed.

In cases of suspected appendicitis, first-choice treatment is surgical consultation and the definitive treatment is emergent appendectomy.[11,23] Surgical intervention is recommended in the first 24 hours in pregnant patients after diagnosis of acute appendicitis to avoid complications, such as perforation.[11] Patients should remain restricted

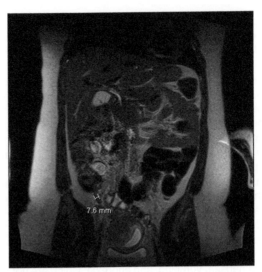

Fig. 3. Appendix measuring 7.6 mm found on MRI during early pregnancy, indicating the diagnosis of appendicitis.

to nothing by mouth and have adequate hydration with intravenous fluids. Preoperative antibiotics to cover gram-negative bacteria and anaerobes are recommended (a second-generation or third-generation cephalosporin or a fluoroquinolone and metronidazole for 7–10 days).[23]

Cholecystitis

After appendicitis, cholecystitis is the second most common surgical condition during pregnancy.[28,29] Acute gallbladder diseases seem to be more common in pregnant women than in nonpregnant women.[30] The incidence of gallstone disease complicating pregnancy is 0.05% to 0.8%.[29] Cholecystitis typically presents as pain in the right upper quadrant or epigastrium and can radiate to the back. It is associated with nausea, vomiting, fever, and the inability to tolerate fatty foods. Initially the pain comes for 30 minutes to 3 hours and then disappears. If the disease progresses to cholecystitis, the pain becomes constant. The differential diagnosis of right upper quadrant abdominal pain is summarized in **Box 2**.

As discussed previously, hormonal changes during pregnancy increase the risk of cholecystitis. An elevated estrogen level causes aggregation of cholesterol crystals and thus leads to increased viscosity of bile and gallstone formation (**Fig. 5**). The other important hormone during pregnancy, progesterone, leads to smooth muscle relaxation and bile sludging, creating a good environment for the development of cholelithiasis.

Signs and symptoms of acute cholecystitis are similar to those in the nonpregnant population: nausea, vomiting, fever, and right upper quadrant pain. Laboratory values are typically not useful, because the white blood cell count, amylase level, and alkaline phosphatase concentration are all elevated during a normal pregnancy. The diagnostic test of choice for all patients with right upper quadrant pain is ultrasound. In addition to being noninvasive and posing no radiation risk to the fetus, ultrasound is 95% to 98% accurate in detecting changes in the gallbladder.[31] The diagnosis of

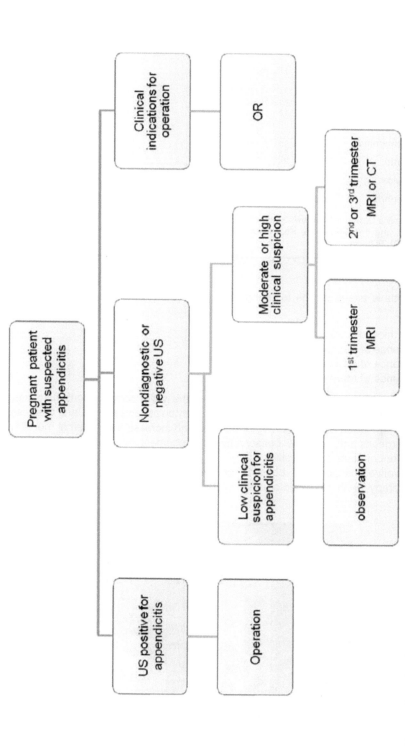

Fig. 4. Algorithm for the evaluation of pregnant patients with suspected appendicitis. OR, operating room; US, ultrasound. (*From* Freeland M, King E, Safcsak K, et al. Diagnosis of appendicitis in pregnancy. Am J Surg 2009;198(6):753–8; with permission.)

> **Box 2**
> **Nonobstetric differential diagnosis of right upper quadrant pain in pregnancy**
>
> - Appendicitis
> - Cholangitis
> - Cholecystitis
> - Cholelithiasis
> - Hepatitis
> - Liver hematoma
> - Pancreatitis
> - Peptic ulcer
> - Pyelonephritis
>
> *Data from* Ma O, Mateer J, Blaivis M. Emergency ultrasound. 2nd edition. New York: McGraw-Hill; 2008; and Benjaminov FS, Heathcote J. Liver disease in pregnancy. Am J Gastroenterol 2004;99(12):2479–88.

cholecystitis is based on the following changes in the gallbladder, as detected by ultrasound[30,31]:

- Wall thickness >3 mm
- Presence of pericholecystic fluid
- Presence of gallstones
- Presence of Murphy sign

If diagnosis and surgical evaluation are delayed, the risk of complications increases. Complications may lead to gallbladder rupture, peritonitis, and sepsis, and they can cause preterm labor, contribute to fetal demise, and increase the maternal mortality rate.[31] Surgeons may choose conservative management or cholecystectomy for management of acute cholecystitis.

Conservative management consists of hydration, supportive care, and anti-biotic therapy with a β-lactamase inhibitor, such as ampicillin-sulbactam,

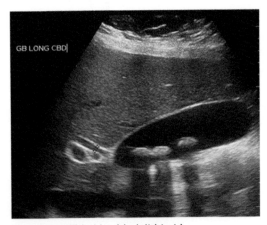

Fig. 5. Gallstones within the gallbladder (cholelithiasis).

piperacillin-tazobactam, or ticarcillin-clavulanate. An alternative antibiotic regimen consists of a third-generation cephalosporin plus metronidazole.[32]

Pancreatitis

Acute pancreatitis complicates as many as 1% of pregnancies (**Box 3**).[33] When pregnancy is complicated by acute pancreatitis, the disease is often mild, self-limited, and managed medically. Pancreatitis most often occurs during the third trimester or immediately postpartum.[1,2,33] This prevalence toward the third trimester is believed to be from increased intra-abdominal pressure from the gravid uterus on the biliary ducts.[1]

The presentation of acute pancreatitis in pregnant women is similar to that in nonpregnant women, involving pain, nausea, vomiting, and fever. Severe preeclampsia can also be a cause of acute pancreatitis because of the microvascular abnormalities that may involve the pancreas, but this is rare.[1]

Once the clinical suspicion for pancreatitis is confirmed with laboratory data, ultrasound becomes the study of choice during pregnancy to determine the cause or contributing complications (**Fig. 6**).[1,2,4,33] Ultrasound can identify common bile duct dilation, cholelithiasis, pancreatic pseudocysts, and abscesses. CT is not indicated unless the course is complicated with severe pancreatitis or extensive necrotic pancreatitis is suspected. MRI can be used to evaluate complications related to pancreatitis, because it provides excellent soft tissue contrast and images of the biliopancreatic duct system (**Fig. 7**).[34]

Management of uncomplicated acute pancreatitis during pregnancy includes supportive care: hospitalization, intravenous fluids, analgesia, and bowel rest.[33] Patients with mild uncomplicated acute pancreatitis and a normal gallbladder do not need antibiotics.[34] Diagnostic endoscopic retrograde cholangiopancreatography should be avoided during pregnancy because of the associated risks (bleeding, perforation, and exposure of fetus to radiation). Gallstone disease is the most common cause of acute pancreatitis during pregnancy. If laparoscopic cholecystectomy is warranted, the second trimester is the preferred time to perform the procedure because of the lower risk of complications to the fetus and only limited technical difficulties from the enlarging uterus.[34]

Adnexal Torsion

Most of the acute causes of abdominal pain discussed in this article are gastrointestinal in nature; the gynecologic system can also have pathology that presents as an acute abdomen. Adnexal torsion complicates 1 in every 1800 pregnancies. Adnexal torsion is a rare occurrence during pregnancy, especially during the third trimester.[33,35] In a patient series studied by Johnson and Woodruff,[35] the incidence was comparable to that of acute appendicitis during pregnancy. This condition is more common during the first and early second trimesters and more often involves the right side.[33,36–38] The incidence increases with ovarian stimulation from assisted reproductive technologies. The rate reaches as high as 6% in those cases and increases to 16% with ovarian hyperstimulation syndrome.[38] Most often the cause of adnexal torsion during pregnancy is the presence of a corpus luteum cyst.[37] Two reasons for the increased incidence on the right have been proposed[37]:

- The right utero-ovarian ligament is longer
- Sigmoid colon on the left reduces space for torsion to occur

The presentation of pregnant and nonpregnant patients with adnexal torsion seems to be similar: most women present with acute onset of sharp lower abdominal pain. The pain can wax and wane for hours to days with or without nausea and vomiting.[4,33]

Box 3
Acute pancreatitis

Presentation of Acute Pancreatitis

- Radiating epigastric pain
  - Back
  - Flank
  - Scapula
- Nausea
- Vomiting
- Fever

Causes of Acute Pancreatitis

- Cholelithiasis
- Alcohol abuse
- Infectious
  - Viral, bacterial, parasitic
- Traumatic
- Hyperlipidemic
- Preeclampsia

Diagnosis of Acute Pancreatitis

- Physical examination
  - Hypoactive bowel sounds
  - Diffuse tenderness
- Abdominal ultrasound
  - Cholelithiasis
  - Bile duct dilation
  - Pancreatic pseudocyst
- Elevated amylase and lipase

Management of Acute Pancreatitis

- Bowel rest
- Rehydration
- Electrolyte repletion
- Analgesia
- Observation
- Antispasmodics

Diagnostic evaluation includes blood work and a pelvic examination to detect an adnexal mass and localized tenderness followed by imaging. In most cases, ultrasound is the preferred modality to image the adnexa. A transabdominal approach can be used initially, with the patient's bladder full. This approach is more useful later in pregnancy, because the ovaries are lifted out of the pelvis by the expanding uterus.[39] If the adnexal structures are not well visualized with that approach, then

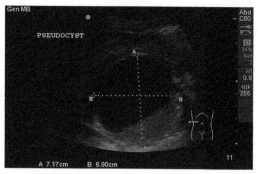

Fig. 6. Ultrasound image of pancreatic pseudocyst.

the transvaginal approach can be used after a patient has emptied her bladder.[37] If adnexal torsion is suspected, Doppler flow should be added to the ultrasound examination. The presence of Doppler flow does not exclude the diagnosis of torsion. That diagnosis is usually revealed at the time of surgery by the physical appearance of the fallopian tube and adnexa.[4] Obstetric consultation should be obtained promptly when torsion is suspected.

Intestinal Obstruction

Intestinal obstructions complicate as many as 1 in 1500 to 3000 pregnancies **(Box 4)**.[2,4,33] They most often occur in the third trimester because of the mechanical effects of the rapidly growing gravid uterus on the gastrointestinal tract.[33] Obstructions also occur in the immediate postpartum period from the rapidly decreasing size of the uterus. Among patients with bowel obstruction, the maternal mortality rate can be as high as 6% and the fetal mortality rate as high as 26%. This risk

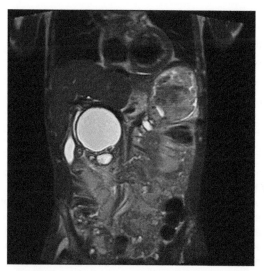

Fig. 7. MRI of the same patient in **Fig. 6**, showing pancreatic pseudocyst at the head of pancreas.

Box 4
Intestinal obstruction

Presentation of Intestinal Obstruction

- Abdominal pain; constant or colicky
  - Every 4–5 minutes with small bowel obstruction
  - Every 10–15 minutes with large bowel obstruction
- Nausea, vomiting, obstipation
- Distended and tympanic abdomen

Causes of Intestinal Obstruction

- Adhesions
  - ↑ Abdominal procedures
  - ↑ Incidence of pelvic inflammatory disease
- Volvulus
- Intussusception
- Hernias
- Neoplasm

Diagnosis of Intestinal Obstruction

- Serial abdominal examinations
- X-ray imaging
  - Supine and upright
- Ultrasound
- Colonoscopy
- CT scan

Management of Intestinal Obstruction

- Decompression
- Intravenous hydration
- Electrolyte repletion
- Surgical evaluation
- Enemas
- Fetal monitoring
- Analgesia

---

increases in the third trimester, when the maternal mortality rate can reach 10% to 20%, especially if the diagnosis is delayed.[1]

The incidence of bowel obstruction increased recently, perhaps because of an increase in the number of abdominal procedures, an increased incidence of pelvic inflammatory disease (both of which increase the risk of adhesions), and an increase in the number of older women becoming pregnant.[33] Adhesions are thought to cause 60% to 70% of small bowel obstructions during pregnancy.[33]

The approach to pregnant patients suspected of having a bowel obstruction is similar to that for nonpregnant patients. A history of bowel obstruction, abdominal surgeries, or pelvic infections or the known presence of hernias should raise a physician's concern about obstruction. The diagnosis is based on the results of serial physical examinations and imaging. The initial imaging approach is an abdominal series of radiographs, which should include supine and upright views.[33] Serial abdominal films obtained at 4-hour to 6-hour intervals showing air-fluid levels or progressive bowel dilation are diagnostic for intestinal obstruction.[1] If radiographs are inconclusive, additional imaging should not be withheld. A CT scan can show an intestinal obstruction of the small bowel. Ultrasound might show a hernia defect if an incarcerated hernia is suspected based on physical examination or patient history. Colonoscopy allows identification and treatment of sigmoid volvulus. Ultimately, evaluation by a surgeon should not be delayed once the diagnosis is suspected.

EMERGENCY DEPARTMENT MANAGEMENT
Imaging

Pregnant patients presenting to an ED create some tension, particularly in regard to imaging. The use of imaging to aid in the diagnosis of pregnant patients with acute abdominal pain has risen in recent years and is a popular topic of debate in the radiology literature.[40] When an emergency physician decides that additional imaging is needed to aid in the diagnosis, then the first choice must be one that exposes the fetus to the least ionizing radiation. Ultrasonography and MRI are thus the preferred modalities. Regardless of which imaging modality is used, physicians should use the principle, as low as reasonably achievable (ALARA). A discussion with a radiologist clarifies which diagnostic test should be done in each clinical case. To help in the decision-making process, radiologists should inform patients of the risks and benefits of the test.

Ultrasound

Ultrasound is considered safe during pregnancy. No adverse fetal outcomes to the fetus from ultrasound exposure have been documented. The use of Doppler ultrasound can produce high intensities; therefore, its use should be limited and, when used, the lowest level possible of acoustic output should be used.[41]

MRI

MRI should be used often to aid in the diagnosis of abdominal pain during pregnancy (**Fig. 8**). Throughout its 20-year history, many studies have not detected adverse fetal outcomes when magnetic field strengths of 1.5 T or lower are used.[41,42] Some concern remains about the effects of heat, radiofrequency pulses, and acoustics on the fetus, so the ALARA principle should be followed.[41–43] The risk of acoustic damage seems theoretic, not actual.[43]

Gadolinium is a category C drug in the classification system of the US Food and Drug Administration; however, no known adverse fetal outcomes have been reported after its intravenous administration.[41,42] Gadolinium crosses the placenta and presumably is excreted by the fetal kidney into the amniotic fluid. It should be avoided in pregnancy and used clinically only if necessary after a discussion with the radiologist and patient about the risks and benefits.[43]

CT

The use of CT imaging during pregnancy has long been a concern, because of the effects of ionizing radiation exposure on the fetus. At times, CT can be used in the work-up of pregnant patients with abdominal pain. Ultrasound imaging might be non-diagnostic or unavailable, and obtaining MRI might significantly delay diagnosis. CT is

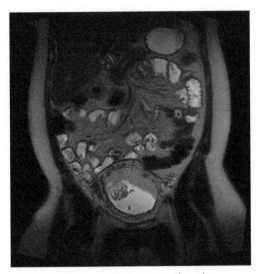

Fig. 8. Gravid uterus as seen with magnetic resonance imaging.

readily available in most EDs and can aid in swift diagnosis when other modalities are nondiagnostic or unavailable. The risk of radiation exposure must be weighed against the effects of a delay in diagnosis. Estimated radiation threshold doses and possible effects on the fetus at different stages of development are presented in **Table 1**.[41,42]

The fetus absorbs 17 mGy to 25 mGy when exposed to a typical CT scan of the abdomen and pelvis.[41] One study that measured the radiation absorbed by the fetus over a 10-year period from abdominal and pelvic CT showed the average estimated fetal dose to be 17.15 mGy.[40] Iodinated intravenous contrast crosses the placenta but has a Food and Drug Administration category B drug rating.[41] Iodinated contrast material has the potential to depress fetal thyroid function, but this risk was not evident in several studies.[41–43] In the United States, thyroid function is tested as part of newborn screening. This practice is particularly important if a mother has a known exposure to intravenous contrast material.

Another concern regarding fetal exposure to ionized radiation is the risk of childhood cancer. There is still much debate about whether or not exposure increases this risk. One study found that the theoretic risk of childhood cancers doubles with exposure to radiation from a CT scan to the abdomen/pelvis as a fetus.[44] According to a policy statement, however, issued by the National Council on Radiation Protection

Table 1		
Effect of ionizing radiation on the fetus		
Gestation Period	**Effects**	**Radiation Dose Threshold**
Implantation: 0–2 wk	Death or no effect	50–100 mGy
Organogenesis: 2–8 wk	Congenital abnormalities	200 mGy
	Growth retardation	200–250 mGy
Fetal period: 8–15 wk	Severe mental retardation	60–500 mGy
	Intellectual deficit	25-Point drop in IQ/Gy
	Microcephaly	200 mGy
Fetal period: 16–25 wk	Mental retardation	250–280 mGy

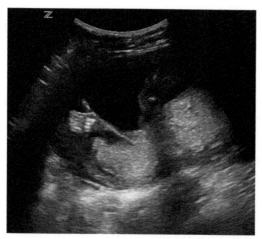

Fig. 9. Do not risk a delayed or missed diagnosis which could cause more harm to the fetus.

and Measurements,[45] "The risk [of abnormality] is considered to be negligible at 50 mGy or less when compared with other risks of pregnancy, and the risk of malformations is significantly increased above control levels only at doses above 150 mGy. Therefore, exposure of the fetus to radiation arising from diagnostic procedures would very rarely because, by itself, for terminating a pregnancy." In summary, obtain the appropriate diagnostic test when the benefit outweighs the risk from a potential delayed or missed diagnosis (**Fig. 9**).

Conventional Radiographs

In the extensive review conducted by Lazarus and colleagues,[40] conventional radiography was the most frequently used imaging modality. The average fetal doses of radiation documented in their study are

- Average for all films: 0.43 mGy
- Fetus in radiation beam (lumbar spine, pelvis, and abdomen): 3.24 mGy
- Fetus not in beam (extremities, chest, head, and cervical and thoracic spine): 0.01 mGy

Plain films can be used to look for intestinal obstruction when spaced several hours apart. They are also used frequently in trauma to evaluate patients for fractures or dislocations. When the abdomen is not the main area to be exposed to an x-ray, a shield can protect the fetus from unnecessary exposure.

SUMMARY

Abdominal pain is common during pregnancy. When a pregnant patient presents to an ED with an abdominal complaint, several dilemmas emerge in association with the evaluation and work-up. Subtle differences in laboratory values need to be acknowledged when assessing patients. Atypical presentations of common diseases can be seen during pregnancy. The prevalence of abdominal disorders varies based on gestational age; for example, bowel obstruction is more common in the third trimester and appendicitis is more common in the second trimester. Emergency physicians should have some degree of hesitancy when deciding which imaging modality to use in pregnant patients. All of these factors can contribute to a delay in diagnosis, increasing the risk of morbidity to mother and fetus. An astute clinician recognizes these changes and promptly evaluates, works-up, and diagnoses pregnant patients presenting with nonobstetric abdominal pain.

REFERENCES

1. Augustin G, Majerovic M. Non-obstetrical acute abdomen during pregnancy. Eur J Obstet Gynecol Reprod Biol 2007;131(1):4–12.
2. Parangi S. Surgical gastrointestinal disorders during pregnancy. Am J Surg 2007; 193(2):223–32.
3. Firstenberg MS, Malangoni MA. Gastrointestinal surgery during pregnancy. Gastroenterol Clin North Am 1998;27(1):73–88.
4. Kilpatrick CC, Monga M. Approach to the acute abdomen in pregnancy. Obstet Gynecol Clin North Am 2007;34(3):389–402, x.
5. Gilstrap LC 3rd, Ramin SM. Urinary tract infections during pregnancy. Obstet Gynecol Clin North Am 2001;28(3):581–91.
6. Nicolle LE. Infectious Diseases Society of America guidelines for the diagnosis and treatment of asymptomatic bacteriuria in adults. Clin Infect Dis 2005;40(5): 643–54.
7. Hill JB. Acute pyelonephritis in pregnancy. Obstet Gynecol 2005;105(1):18–23.
8. Sharma P, Thapa L. Acute pyelonephritis in pregnancy: a retrospective study. Aust N Z J Obstet Gynaecol 2007;47(4):313–5.
9. Cavorsi K, Prabhakar P, Kirby C. Acute Pyelonephritis. Ultrasound Q 2010;26(2): 103–5.
10. Ueberrueck T. Ninety-four appendectomies for suspected acute appendicitis during pregnancy. World J Surg 2004;28(5):508–11.
11. Murariu D. Case report and management of suspected acute appendicitis. Hawaii Med J 2011;70:30–2.
12. Wittich AC, DeSantis RA, Lockrow EG. Appendectomy during pregnancy: a survey of two army medical activities. Mil Med 1999;164(10):671–4.
13. Somani RA. Appendicitis in pregnancy: a rare presentation. CMAJ 2003;168(8): 1020.
14. Gilo NB, Amini D, Landy HJ. Appendicitis and cholecystitis in pregnancy. Clin Obstet Gynecol 2009;52(4):586–96.
15. Guttman R, Goldman R, Koren G. Appendicitis during pregnancy. Can Fam Physician 2004;50:355–7.
16. Carlin A, Alfirevic Z. Physiological changes of pregnancy and monitoring. Best Pract Res Clin Obstet Gynaecol 2008;22(5):801–23.
17. Mourad J. Appendicitis in pregnancy: new information that contradicts long-held clinical beliefs. Am J Obstet Gynecol 2000;182(5):1027–9.
18. Hodjati H, Kazerooni T. Location of the appendix in the gravid patient: a re-evaluation of the established concept. Int J Gynaecol Obstet 2003;81(3):245–7.
19. Yilmaz HG. Acute appendicitis in pregnancy—risk factors associated with principal outcomes: a case control study. Int J Surg 2007;5(3):192–7.
20. Vu L. Evaluation of MRI for the diagnosis of appendicitis during pregnancy when ultrasound is inconclusive. J Surg Res 2009;156(1):145–9.
21. Long SS. Imaging strategies for right lower quadrant pain in pregnancy. AJR Am J Roentgenol 2011;196(1):4–12.
22. Freeland M. Diagnosis of appendicitis in pregnancy. Am J Surg 2009;198(6):753–8.
23. Vissers RJ, Lennarz WB. Pitfalls in appendicitis. Emerg Med Clin North Am 2010; 28(1):103–18, viii.

24. Cobben L. MRI for clinically suspected appendicitis during pregnancy. AJR Am J Roentgenol 2004;183:671–5.
25. Pedrosa I. MR imaging evaluation of acute appendicitis in pregnancy. Radiology 2006;238(3):891–9.
26. Oto A. MR imaging in the triage of pregnant patients with acute abdominal and pelvic pain. Abdom Imaging 2009;34(2):243–50.
27. Singh AK, Desai H, Novelline RA. Emergency MRI of acute pelvic pain: MR protocol with no oral contrast. Emerg Radiol 2009;16(2):133–41.
28. Ghumman E, Barry M, Grace PA. Management of gallstones in pregnancy. Br J Surg 1997;84(12):1646–50.
29. Date RS, Kaushal M, Ramesh A. A review of the management of gallstone disease and its complications in pregnancy. Am J Surg 2008;196(4):599–608.
30. Ma O, Mateer J, Blaivis M. Emergency ultrasound. 2nd edition. New York: Mcgraw-Hill; 2008.
31. Tseng JY. Acute cholecystitis during pregnancy: what is the best approach? Taiwan J Obstet Gynecol 2009;48(3):305–7.
32. Brooks D. Gallstone disease in pregnant women. Wolters Kluwer Health; 2012.
33. Cappell MS, Friedel D. Abdominal pain during pregnancy. Gastroenterol Clin North Am 2003;32(1):1–58.
34. Pitchumoni CS, Yegneswaran B. Acute pancreatitis in pregnancy. World J Gastroenterol 2009;15(45):5641–6.
35. Johnson TR Jr, Woodruff JD. Surgical emergencies of the uterine adnexae during pregnancy. Int J Gynaecol Obstet 1986;24(5):331–5.
36. Prefumo F, Ciravolo G. Adnexal torsion in late pregnancy. Arch Gynecol Obstet 2009;280:473–4.
37. Huchon C, Fauconnier A. Adnexal torsion: a literature review. Eur J Obstet Gynecol Reprod Biol 2010;150(1):8–12.
38. Hasson J. Comparison of adnexal torsion between pregnant and nonpregnant women. Am J Obstet Gynecol 2010;202(6):536.e1–6.
39. Graham L, American College of, and Gynecologists. ACOG releases guidelines on management of adnexal masses. Am Fam Physician 2008;77(9):1320–3.
40. Lazarus E. Utilization of imaging in pregnant patients: 10-year review of 5270 examinations in 3285 patients–1997-2006. Radiology 2009;251(2):517–24.
41. Katz DS. Imaging of abdominal pain in pregnancy. Radiol Clin North Am 2012;50(1):149–71.
42. Patel SJ. Imaging the pregnant patient for nonobstetric conditions: algorithms and radiation dose considerations. Radiographics 2007;27(6):1705–22.
43. Chen MM. Guidelines for computed tomography and magnetic resonance imaging use during pregnancy and lactation. Obstet Gynecol 2008;112(2 Pt 1):333–40.
44. Hurwitz LM. Radiation dose to the fetus from body MDCT during early gestation. AJR Am J Roentgenol 2006;186(3):871–6.
45. National Council on Radiation Protection and Measurements. Medical radiation exposure of pregnant and potentially pregnant women. NCRP report no. 54. Bethesda (MD): National Council on Radiation Protection and Measurements; 1977.

Hypertension and Pregnancy

Teresa M. Deak, MD[a], Joshua B. Moskovitz, MD, MPH[a,b,*]

KEYWORDS

- Pregnancy • Pregnant • Preeclampsia • Eclampsia • Hypertension • Hypertensive
- Hypertensive crisis • Hypertensive emergency

KEY POINTS

- Mild hypertension in pregnancy without end-organ damage does not require treatment.
- Hypertension above 150/100 mm Hg or evidence of end-organ damage requires treatment, because maternal and fetal morbidity and mortality rates increase.
- Physicians should use the antihypertensive agent with which they feel most comfortable when treating pregnant patients, because there is little evidence to suggest which is superior.
- Severe gestational hypertension has more adverse outcomes than mild preeclampsia.
- The progression of preeclampsia to eclampsia is sudden and without prediction. Patients with this condition should be admitted for observation.

INTRODUCTION

Hypertensive disorders of pregnancy complicate 1% of gestations[1] and account for 16% of maternal deaths,[2] making it vital to obtain accurate blood pressure (BP) measurements. During pregnancy, normal physiologic changes are reflected in the BP, which is a product of cardiac output multiplied by systemic vascular resistance. Systemic vascular resistance decreases because of rising levels of progesterone, resulting in a decrease in BP during the first 16 to 18 weeks of gestation (WGA). At 36 weeks, BP increases to prepregnancy levels and is expected to rise after delivery. Furthermore, there is a large increase in cardiac output and intravascular volume, with resultant increase in renal plasma flow and glomerular filtration rate. In the nonemergent patient, BP measurements should be taken at least 4 hours apart but no more than 7 days apart to establish the diagnosis.[1]

No financial disclosures or conflicts of interest.
[a] Department of Emergency Medicine, North Shore University Hospital, 300 Community Drive, Manhasset, NY 11030, USA; [b] Department of Emergency Medicine, Hofstra North Shore-LIJ School of Medicine, 1000 Fulton Avenue, Hempstead, NY 11549, USA
* Corresponding author. Department of Emergency Medicine, North Shore University Hospital, 300 Community Drive, Manhasset, NY 11030.
E-mail address: joshmoskovitz@gmail.com

Emerg Med Clin N Am 30 (2012) 903–917
http://dx.doi.org/10.1016/j.emc.2012.08.006
emed.theclinics.com

CHRONIC HYPERTENSION

Definition

In nonpregnant patients, chronic hypertension or preexisting hypertension is defined as an elevated BP. The parameters are a systolic BP greater than 140 mm Hg or a diastolic BP greater than 90 mm Hg on two occasions before 20 WGA or persisting longer than 12 weeks postpartum.

Chronic hypertension can be difficult to diagnose if the BP before 16 WGA is unknown because there are normal physiologic changes in BP during the first trimester.[3,4] Prepregnancy BP normally returns in the third trimester, with persistently elevated BP beyond 12 weeks postpartum confirming the diagnosis of chronic hypertension.

Chronic hypertension is divided into two categories: primary (or essential; 90%) and secondary (10%).[5] Young women with preexisting hypertension or early gestational diabetes are more likely to have secondary hypertension (**Table 1**). Further testing should be based on suspicion of a secondary cause of hypertension.[1]

Chronic hypertension in pregnancy is also categorized according to severity as either mild (systolic pressure of 140–159 mm Hg or diastolic pressure of 90–109 mm Hg) or severe (systolic >160 mm Hg or diastolic >100 mm Hg).[3,6] Women with mild uncomplicated primary hypertension with no end-organ involvement are considered to be at low risk for adverse complications.[7]

Pathophysiology

The prevalence of primary and secondary hypertension has increased over the past decade, with primary hypertension increasing from 0.09% in 1995 to 1996 to 1.52% in 2007 to 2008.[5] This could be secondary to increases in maternal age, obesity, and type 2 diabetes mellitus.[4] The prevalence of secondary hypertension increased from 0.07% in 1995 to 1996 to 0.24% in 2007 to 2008.[5]

Chronic hypertension during pregnancy increases the risk of maternal and fetal morbidity and mortality. Superimposed preeclampsia, maternal mortality, cerebrovascular accident, pulmonary edema, and renal failure all carry odds ratios greater than five compared with pregnant women who are normotensive.[4,5,8–11] Risks also increase for cesarean section, postpartum hemorrhage, placental abruption, preterm labor, small for gestation age, and neonatal mortality (**Table 2**). Women with chronic hypertension and baseline proteinuria early in pregnancy are also at increased risk

Table 1 Assessment of secondary hypertension in pregnancy	
Causes of Secondary Hypertension	**Suggestive Signs and Symptoms**
Pheochromocytoma	Palpitations, paroxysmal hypertension, panic attacks, sweating, headaches
Cushing syndrome	Moon facies, central obesity
Renal artery stenosis	<30 years of age, severe hypertension, renal bruit
Coarctation of aorta	Delayed or absent femoral pulses
Chronic renal disease	
Hyperaldosteronism	Low potassium
Hyperthyroid	Hyperthermia, hyperreflexia, tachycardia

Data from References.[3–5,18,20]

Table 2 Maternal and fetal complications in chronic hypertension	
Complication	Odds Ratio
Cesarean section	3
Postpartum hemorrhage	2
Placental abruption	2[a]
Small for gestational age	2–5
Neonatal mortality	2–4

[a] Present in 8.4% of patients with severe hypertension.
Data from References.[3–5,8,9,11,12,40]

for adverse neonatal outcomes, including preterm delivery and small gestational age, compared with women with chronic hypertension alone.[4,12]

Management

Preferably, the evaluation of chronic hypertension begins before the patient becomes pregnant, directed at determining its cause and severity, including evidence of end-organ damage. An obstetric history includes maternal and neonatal outcomes of previous pregnancies, including abruptio placentae, preeclampsia, preterm delivery, and small-for-gestational-age infants. Initial laboratory tests include a complete blood count, a basic metabolic panel, urinalysis, urine culture, 24-hour urine protein, and glucose tolerance testing.[3,4] In women with a long history of hypertension, a more thorough evaluation for end-organ damage should be pursued. In this subset of patients, testing includes ophthalmologic examination; creatinine clearance; and an electrocardiogram, and if abnormal, an echocardiogram.[1,4,11]

Treatment for chronic hypertension depends on the severity of disease. Mild hypertension has similar maternal and fetal outcomes as in the general population.[3,4,13] Although treatment decreases the risk of severe maternal hypertension, there is no change in maternal or fetal outcome.[3,4,13] In addition, evidence suggests antihypertensive treatment decreases mean arterial pressure and impairs fetal growth.[14] Because the treatment of mild hypertension does not demonstrate decreases in rates of preterm delivery, preeclampsia, or abruptio placentae,[1,3,4,13] tapering or discontinuing antihypertensive medicine with close observation is appropriate.[1,3,4,15] Treatment is initiated if the BP rises above 150/100 mm Hg or if the patient has end-organ damage.[3]

Fetal assessment in women with mild chronic hypertension starts with an ultrasound examination at 18 to 20 WGA, repeated monthly until delivery.[1,4] If fetal growth restriction is suspected based on the ultrasound image, a nonstress test or biophysical profile should be completed.[1,3] In the setting of mild chronic hypertension with no evidence of fetal growth restriction, delivery should be expected at 38 to 40 WGA.[3,4]

Emergency Department Presentation

Patients with severe hypertension are at increased risk of maternal and fetal complications; therefore, treatment is mandated.[3,4] Stroke is one of the most serious maternal complications of hypertension during pregnancy, accounting for 5% of maternal deaths,[16] with systolic BP greater than 160 mm Hg being an independent risk factor.[17] Treatment is imperative, because it reduces the incidence of stroke.[3] Consensus in the United States is that a pregnant woman with BP greater than 150 to 160/100 to 110 mm Hg should be treated with medications.[15] Lowering the BP lowers the mean arterial pressure, which may lead to small gestational age.[14] The goal for BP is less than 150 to 160/100 mm Hg[11,18–20] unless end-organ damage is noted. Then, the recommendation of the American Congress of Obstetricians and Gynecologists is systolic pressure less than 140 mm Hg and diastolic pressure less than 90 mm Hg.[3] Laboratory tests should be monitored more closely in these patients than in those with mild hypertension.

A woman with uncontrolled hypertension may require hospitalization to regain BP control and assess for end-organ damage,[4] although this scenario is rare.[6] Visual symptoms and headaches, although they can be serious, have a low incidence of adverse central nervous system outcomes.[6] Management is similar to that of the general population, with initial reduction of 25% during the first hour and then further reduction over hours to a goal of less than 160/100 mm Hg.[1,6,15]

An increase in fetal assessment intervals in severe hypertension is necessary to look for common complications, such as small gestational age. Ultrasound imaging should be performed between 18 and 20 WGA, at 28 WGA, and then every 3 weeks until delivery.[4] If the fetus is found to have fetal growth restriction, hospitalization may be indicated.[4] A nonstress test or biophysical profile should be performed at 28 WGA and then weekly until delivery.[4,20] If BP is well controlled with medication, then delivery proceeds at 37 to 39 WGA.[1] If the hypertension is difficult to control, delivery should be at 36 to 37 WGA,[1,4] with consideration of delivery at 34 WGA in the advent of complications, such as small gestational age.[4]

Women with chronic hypertension have increased risk of postpartum complications, including pulmonary edema, hypertensive encephalopathy, and renal failure.[1,4] Those with cardiac disease, with chronic renal disease, and taking multiple antihypertensive agents are at even higher risk.[1] Women should be observed for 48 hours postpartum for these complications.[4]

Emergency Department Management

Treating hypertension in pregnancy requires an efficacious drug that is tolerated well by the patient while posing the least risk to the fetus. Of the drugs considered safe, there are limited data demonstrating which is most efficacious. Physicians should use the medications with which they are most comfortable and that are safe for the fetus.[21]

Methyldopa, a centrally acting α_2-adrenergic agonist, has traditionally been used to treat hypertension in pregnancy, with no adverse maternal or fetal outcomes.[4] A follow-up study of neonates exposed to methyldopa, conducted when they were 7.5 years of age, showed normal intelligence and neurocognitive development.[3,4,22] The starting dose is 250 mg twice daily, with a maximum of 4 g daily.[4] The side effects that limit the use of this medication are maternal sedation and fatigue.[3] Methyldopa is also safe for breastfeeding mothers.

Labetalol, an α/β-blocker, has become one of the first-line drugs for treatment,[3,4,23] because there are no known adverse maternal or fetal outcomes.[4,15] Oral dosing starts at 100 mg twice daily, with a maximum of 2400 mg daily.[4] In a hypertensive urgency or emergency, a 20- to 40-mg intravenous bolus every 10 to 15 minutes can be administered, with a maximum of 220 mg.[4] Labetalol is also safe during breastfeeding,[20] but it should be avoided in women with asthma and congestive heart failure.[15] Atenolol has been associated with fetal growth restriction and therefore is not recommended in pregnancy.[3,4]

Calcium channel blockers can be used safely in pregnancy, because nifedipine demonstrated no adverse fetal outcomes on development 1.5 years after delivery.[4] For maintenance, nifedipine is started at 10 mg twice daily, with a maximum of 120 mg daily.[4] In uncontrolled hypertension, it is administered at doses of 10 to 20 mg by mouth every 30 minutes, with a maximum of 50 mg.[4]

The smooth muscle relaxer hydralazine may be associated with increased maternal hypotension and adverse fetal heart rate.[6] Also associated with reflex tachycardia, flushing, and headaches,[20] it is safe in lactating patients. During hypertensive crisis, it is given as 5 to 10 mg intravenously every 20 minutes, to a maximum of 30 mg.[4]

Thiazides are the most commonly used diuretics. They are associated with decreased plasma volume, although there are no associated adverse effects.[3,4,20] Diuretics are not to be used in patients with diabetes and should be stopped if the patient develops preeclampsia or fetal growth restriction.[4] Thiazide diuretics are started at 12.5 mg by mouth twice daily, with a maximum of 50 mg daily.[4]

Angiotensin-converting enzyme inhibitors are not safe in pregnancy[3] because they are associated with major congenital malformations when given in the first trimester.[24] Most heavily associated with cardiovascular and central nervous system malformations,[24] they have been demonstrated to cause oligohydramnios and fetal-neonatal renal failure.[4] However, captopril and enalapril are safe during breastfeeding.[20]

Nitroprusside, although not a first-line agent, is sometimes used in hypertensive emergencies when other medications fail to control hypertension. There is a theoretic risk of cyanide poisoning if used longer than 4 hours.[15] An infusion can be started at 0.25 to 5 μg/kg/min.[15]

GESTATIONAL HYPERTENSION
Definition

Gestational hypertension is hypertension associated with pregnancy and resolves after delivery. It is identified when a patient who is normotensive before 20 WGA develops a systolic BP greater than 140 mm Hg or a diastolic BP greater than 90 mm Hg on two occasions after 20 WGA. Severe gestational hypertension is defined as systolic BP greater than 160 mm Hg and diastolic BP greater than 110 mm Hg. If the patient remains hypertensive more than 12 weeks postpartum, then she is reclassified as having chronic hypertension.

Gestational hypertension complicates 6% to 7% of pregnancies.[25,26] Diabetes, cardiac disease, renal disease, advanced maternal age, obesity, and multiple gestations all increase the risk of gestational hypertension.[25,26] Women with a history of preeclampsia have a risk of 11% for developing mild gestational hypertension and a 4% risk of developing severe gestational hypertension.[25,27]

Women with gestational hypertension are at an increased risk of preterm delivery, preeclampsia, and abruptio placentae,[25] with higher rates of small gestational age and neonatal morbidity in infants delivered between 35 and 37 WGA.[28] Severe gestational hypertension has more adverse perinatal outcomes (preterm delivery and small gestational age) than mild preeclampsia.[27] In addition, severe gestational hypertension has similar perinatal outcomes as severe preeclampsia.[27] Women with gestational hypertension frequently develop hypertension later in life.[25]

Emergency Department Management

Patients diagnosed with gestational hypertension should have initial testing for preeclampsia, including a complete blood count, a comprehensive metabolic panel, urine microanalysis, 24-hour urine protein, and measurement of lactate dehydrogenase (LDH). A nonstress test and ultrasound examination for fetal weight and amniotic fluid index should be performed to look for small gestational age. There is no need to repeat a nonstress test or biophysical profile unless there is a change in maternal condition, decreased fetal movement, or abnormal fundal height. Laboratory tests are repeated weekly and include a complete blood count, a comprehensive metabolic panel, and 24-hour urine protein. In addition, BP should be checked every other week, with a urine dip and assessment for symptoms of preeclampsia. If there is a change in symptoms or an elevation in BP, the patient needs further evaluation for preeclampsia.[29]

In mild gestational hypertension, the maternal and fetal outcomes are similar to those in the general population.[27] Women with mild gestational hypertension are not treated with antihypertensive medications but are observed for progression of the disease. In contrast, severe gestational hypertension is treated with antihypertensive medications. There are insufficient data to support a target BP[30]; therefore, the same guidelines for BP control in chronic hypertension in pregnancy are used for gestational hypertension. Antihypertensive medications can be discontinued 3 to 4 weeks postpartum.[1]

In controlled gestational hypertension, delivery is at 37 to 38 WGA to limit progression of maternal disease without increasing neonatal morbidity.[31,32] If delivery occurs at 40 WGA, the risk of cesarean delivery and neonatal morbidities increases.[32] In women with gestational hypertension between 34 and 37 WGA, expectant management can be pursued. However, with severe hypertension, vaginal bleeding, abnormal fetal testing, preterm labor, or rupture of membranes, delivery should be performed.[32]

PREECLAMPSIA
Definition

Preeclampsia is a constellation of symptoms thought to be caused by inflammation, with the pathophysiology largely unknown. It starts with incomplete trophoblast invasion into the endometrium, causing inadequate placental implantation. This causes decreased angiogenic growth factor and increased placental debris in the maternal circulation, resulting in maternal inflammation of the endothelium and cardiovascular system.[20] The endothelial inflammation increases vascular reactivity and disrupts sodium volume homeostasis, reversing the natural cardiovascular changes of pregnancy.[2]

Every organ system is affected by preeclampsia. Decreased cardiac output and decreased arterial compliance result in hypertension[11] and activation of the coagulation system, manifesting most commonly as thrombocytopenia with increased platelet activation and decreased platelet lifespan.

Preeclampsia is defined as gestational hypertension plus proteinuria. The gold standard is a 24-urine protein of at least 300 mg[29]; however, 24-hour urine tests are frequently inaccurate because undercollection and overcollection.[33] On urinalysis, 1+ protein is commonly used as an indicator of preeclampsia.[1,11] Urine dipped for protein can yield false-positive and false-negative results secondary to variable excretion, maternal dehydration, or bacteriuria and are not the most consistent, but this test is used because it is so easily accessible. The urine creatinine/protein ratio can be calculated to evaluate for proteinuria (with a value >0.3 mg/mmol considered indicative), though its accuracy is still being investigated.[11]

Preeclampsia is classified as mild if the systolic BP is less than 160 mm Hg or the diastolic BP is less than 110 mm Hg with normal platelets and liver enzymes and absence of cerebral symptoms. Preeclampsia is classified as severe if the systolic BP is greater than 160 mm Hg or the diastolic BP is greater than 110 mm. Severe preeclampsia can also be classified by proteinuria greater than 5 g in 24 hours; greater than 3+ protein on two occasions, 3 hours apart; or oliguria (<500 mL in 24 hours) (Table 3). Thrombocytopenia, impaired liver function, fetal growth restriction, and

Table 3 Classification of preeclampsia		
Mild	Systolic <160 mm Hg	Diastolic <110 mm Hg
	Absence of other symptoms	
Severe	Systolic >160 mm Hg	Diastolic >110 mm Hg
	Proteinuria >5 g/24 h or 3+ microanalysis	Oliguria
	Thrombocytopenia	Impaired liver function
	Cerebral symptoms	Vision changes
	Right upper quadrant pain	Pulmonary edema
	Intrauterine growth restriction	

Data from Leeman L, Fontaine P. Hypertensive disorders of pregnancy. Am Fam Physician 2008;78: 93–100.

pulmonary edema are also indicative of severe disease. Epigastric pain, right upper quadrant pain, visual symptoms, or cerebral symptoms are additional indicators of severe disease.[34]

Preeclampsia complicates 2.2% to 6.3% of pregnancies[2,25,27,35] and is increasing in incidence.[2] Risk factors include diabetes, cardiac disease, renal disease, extremes of maternal age,[36] obesity,[27,36–38] nulliparity,[20,37,39] and multiple gestations.[25,37] Other risk factors include decreased socioeconomic status[2] and prior preeclampsia (7.5%–10% increased risk).[25,27,36,37] Postpartum preeclampsia occurs within 6 weeks after delivery in 5% of patients.[35] Most women with this condition are African American and carry no previous diagnosis of hypertension.[35]

Globally, preeclampsia is the leading cause of maternal and perinatal morbidity and mortality.[2] Associated with stroke, liver rupture,[2] and placental abruption,[29,40] preeclampsia carries an increased risk of preterm delivery,[25] small for gestational age,[2,29] and fetal mortality. When the onset of preeclampsia is before 32 WGA, the maternal mortality rate rises.[2]

Research exploring preeclampsia prevention has been conflicting. A Cochrane Review demonstrated that low-dose aspirin had a moderate benefit in prevention[37,38,41,42] but required a large number needed to treat. There were no differences in outcome when aspirin was started later[41]; therefore, some authors suggest starting aspirin at the beginning of the second trimester.[20] There is no evidence recommending the optimal dose of aspirin or who would benefit most from treatment.

The role of calcium has been investigated in the prevention of preeclampsia with no evidence to support giving supplemental calcium to all pregnant women[1,43]; however, among women with low dietary calcium, there may be some benefit.[11,37,38] Magnesium, omega fatty acids, and antioxidant vitamins have been studied without indication of preventative benefit.[44]

Emergency Department Management

Initial evaluation of the potential preeclamptic patient includes a complete blood count; a comprehensive metabolic panel; urinalysis; 24-hour urine protein assessment; measurement of uric acid, LDH, D dimer, and fibrinogen levels; and coagulation studies. These tests determine the occurrence and severity of the disease (**Table 4**).[2] Fetal testing should include a nonstress test and fetal ultrasound scan, looking for fetal distress, growth restriction, and oligohydramnios.[45]

The progression of preeclampsia is rapid, and hospitalization is usually necessary for the initial evaluation. For mild preeclampsia, monitoring BP without the use of

Table 4
Laboratory assessment in preeclampsia

Labs	Expected Findings
Hemoglobin/hematocrit	Hemoconcentration
Platelets	Thrombocytopenia
Lactate dehydrogenase	Elevated from hemolysis
Uric acid	Elevated
Transaminases	Elevated

Data from Steegers EA, von Dadelszen P, Duvekot JJ, et al. Pre-eclampsia. Lancet 2010;376:631–44.

antihypertensive agents is appropriate, because maternal and fetal outcomes are similar to those associated with mild gestational hypertension.[27] Antihypertensive medicine is started in patients with severe preeclampsia,[29] with a goal BP of 140 to 155 mm Hg systolic and 90 to 105 mm Hg diastolic.[29] Labetalol, hydralazine, and nifedipine are drugs of choice for acute hypertension in preeclampsia. Diuretics should be avoided because patients already are depleted in intravascular volume.

Magnesium in severe preeclampsia prevents disease progression to eclampsia but the evidence in mild preeclampsia is unclear. Although magnesium decreases the risk of progression to eclampsia in half, it does not decrease perinatal morbidity or mortality.[20,43,46] Magnesium reduces the risk of maternal death and recurrent seizures better than diazepam or phenytoin[47,48] and should be initiated 2 hours before elective cesarean delivery and continued for 12 to 24 hours after delivery.[29] A 4-g loading dose of magnesium is given over 10 to 15 minutes followed by an infusion of 1 g/h. If a breakthrough seizure occurs, a second loading dose of 2 to 4 g is given. Continuous infusions may be increased up to 2 g/h as needed while monitoring for toxicity (**Box 1**).[2] If toxicity is noted, calcium gluconate should be given. Shortened postpartum periods of magnesium are currently being studied to determine the minimal amount of time required to be effective. A 6- or 12-hour postpartum regimen followed by 24 hours of observation has been proposed as a safe alternative to 24 hours of postpartum magnesium.[49,50]

Delivery is the definitive treatment for preeclampsia. Although delivery is beneficial for the patient, it is delayed to allow the fetus to mature. Timing of delivery is determined by the condition of the patient, gestational age, evidence of fetal lung maturity, and fetal compromise. In mild preeclampsia, the goal is delivery at 37 WGA,[31,32] because there is no increase in neonatal morbidity and it reduces the risk of progression of disease in the mother.[32,51]

Box 1
Signs of magnesium toxicity

Elevated serum creatinine

Delayed deep tendon reflexes

Decreased urine output

Decreased respiratory drive

Data from Leeman L, Fontaine P. Hypertensive disorders of pregnancy. Am Fam Physician 2008;78:93–100.

In patients at 34 to 37 WGA with mild preeclampsia, expectant management is pursued for the theoretic benefit of improving perinatal outcomes without increasing maternal or fetal risks.[51] Reassuring signs include mild hypertension, absence of preterm labor or rupture of membranes, and no vaginal bleeding.[29] The results of fetal testing should also be normal without evidence of fetal growth restriction, oligohydramnios, variable or late decelerations, or biophysical profile less than six.[29,32] Once the patient no longer meets the criteria for expectant management, delivery is pursued.

Because the severity of BP[52] and proteinuria[45] are not predictive, the fullPIERS (Preeclampsia Integrated Estimate of Risk) model has been developed as a possible predictive rule for adverse maternal outcomes; however, it is quite cumbersome and not geared toward emergency medicine.[53] Evidence suggests that admission uric acid levels are inversely related to the length of expectant management.[54]

In severe, resistant hypertension, intravenous medication is necessary. If cerebral symptoms persist after maximal administration of labetalol, nifedipine, and magnesium, delivery is necessary within 24 to 48 hours regardless of gestational age.[29] Between 24 and 34 WGA, expectant management is associated with decreased perinatal morbidity[45] and perinatal mortality,[51] making it an appropriate choice in selected cases. Delivery is indicated in women with imminent eclampsia, new-onset renal dysfunction, disseminated intravascular coagulation, multiorgan dysfunction, uncontrollable severe hypertension, severe fetal growth restriction, abruptio placentae, or nonreassuring fetal test results.[29,45] Corticosteroids are administered for fetal lung maturity for all pregnancies less than 34 WGA to decrease respiratory distress syndrome, intraventricular hemorrhage, and perinatal mortality.[45] If a patient has severe preeclampsia before 24 WGA, the pregnancy is often terminated because its continuation is unlikely to improve perinatal outcomes and increases maternal risks.[2,51,55,56]

Vaginal delivery can be accomplished in most cases if patients are monitored closely for progression of preeclampsia and need for emergent cesarean section.[29] Cesarean section should be pursued as the initial delivery method in patients with severe preeclampsia less than 30 WGA with a Bishop score less than 5 (**Table 5**)[29] and in those with severe preeclampsia with fetal growth restriction less than 32 WGA with an unfavorable cervical Bishop score.[29]

Postpartum preeclampsia is receiving more attention lately because patients with this condition have an increased risk of pulmonary edema and severe hypertension. Administration of magnesium sulfate for 24 hours, the use of antihypertensive medicines as needed, and consideration of brain imaging[29] are a part of the common treatment algorithm. Late postpartum preeclampsia develops more than 48 hours after delivery.

Even though hypertension usually resolves within 2 to 4 weeks[1] and definitely resolves by 12 weeks postpartum, women who have preeclampsia have an increased

Table 5 Bishop score				
	0	1	2	3
Consistency	Firm	Intermediate	Soft	—
Dilation	0 cm	1–2 cm	3–4 cm	>5 cm
Effacement	0%–30%	31%–50%	51%–80%	>80%
Fetal station	−3	−2	−1, 0	+1, +2
Position	Posterior	Intermediate	Anterior	—

lifetime risk of cardiovascular death.[20] Later in life, they have an increased risk of cardiovascular disease,[2] hypertension, hyperlipidemia, and diabetes.[20]

ECLAMPSIA
Definition

Eclampsia is classically thought of as a progression of preeclampsia; however, evidence suggests this is not true. In one study, a third of patients with eclampsia were not hypertensive before their seizure[57]; therefore, a more appropriate definition of eclampsia is preeclampsia with a seizure.

Eclampsia complicates 5 to 12 cases per 10,000 deliveries in developed countries.[58] Independent risk factors for eclampsia include nulliparity, maternal age, and gestational hypertension.[57]

Emergency Department Management

As with all patients in the emergency department, it is vital to evaluate and appropriately manage the airway and breathing in these patients. Supplemental oxygen is required in patients who are hypoxic and recommended in seizing patients, and airway control as necessary. Hypertensive emergencies and urgencies require parenteral medication and admission to an intensive care setting, with judicious use of intravenous fluid because of the risk of pulmonary edema in these patients. Early obstetric consultation is paramount.

Magnesium is the drug of choice to prevent recurrent seizures and has been demonstrated to be more effective than phenytoin and diazepam.[46] Dosing of magnesium is based on general consensus, with little evidence to support optimal schedules. Four to 6 g are administered intravenously over 15 minutes followed by 2 or 3 g/h, stopping if signs of toxicity emerge. Patients with persistent seizures despite magnesium therapy receive a 2-g bolus over 15 minutes. If the seizure persists, use a traditional antiseizure medicine, such as diazepam or lorazepam.

Delivery is the definitive therapy for eclampsia regardless of gestational age. Vaginal delivery can be attempted; however, women remote from term with an unfavorable cervix often require a cesarean section.

HELLP SYNDROME
Definition

The HELLP syndrome (hemolysis, elevated liver enzyme levels, and low platelet counts) often occurs in pregnant women with preeclampsia or eclampsia; however, the exact relationship between these disease processes is controversial. This syndrome complicates 1 or 2 pregnancies per 1000 and 5% of women with preeclampsia.[11] Associated with maternal and fetal morbidity and mortality, associated problems include pulmonary edema, acute renal failure, liver failure, sepsis, stroke, and acute reactive airway disease. Fetal morbidity includes preterm delivery and small gestational age.[59]

Emergency Department Management

Symptoms of HELLP syndrome vary greatly. Patients often present with abdominal complaints, including pain, tenderness in the right upper quadrant or epigastrium, nausea, vomiting, and jaundice. Headaches and visual changes can also be presenting symptoms. Concern for HELLP syndrome should prompt laboratory analysis, including a complete blood count, a peripheral smear, LDH, and a comprehensive metabolic panel. On peripheral smear, there is evidence of hemolysis with abnormal

Table 6 HELLP syndrome classification scheme	
Class 1	Platelets <50
Class 2	Platelets 50–100
Class 3	Platelets 100–150

erythrocytes. LDH is elevated; serum bilirubin is greater than or equal to 1.2 mg/dL, and the platelet count is less than 100,000/mm^3 with a classification scheme based on platelet count (**Table 6**). Expectant management of HELLP syndrome at less than 34 WGA is associated with increased maternal morbidity but a reduction in neonatal mortality[51]; therefore, patients in this scenario are not typically managed expectantly.[45] In patients at greater than 34 WGA, with severe disease (eg, multiorgan dysfunction, abruptio placenta, or nonreassuring fetal testing), delivery should be initiated promptly. Consider platelet transfusion if there is significant maternal bleeding, if the platelet count is less than 20,000/mm^3, or if a patient with a platelet count less than 40,000/mm^3 is undergoing cesarean delivery. If delivery is occurring at less than 34 WGA, glucocorticoids should be administered to mature fetal lungs. Dexamethasone was initially thought to be beneficial in the HELLP syndrome; however, a review demonstrated no benefit to this practice.[60] After delivery, symptoms usually resolve quickly but may persist for a week.

FATTY LIVER OF PREGNANCY

Acute fatty liver of pregnancy is the infiltration of hepatocytes by microvesicular fat. It complicates 1 in 7000 to 20,000 deliveries. The typical presentation begins with nausea or vomiting, abdominal pain, and jaundice. Initial laboratory assessment includes a complete blood count, a comprehensive metabolic panel, coagulation studies, and LDH. Liver enzymes are elevated along with bilirubin levels, and sometimes the platelet count is decreased. Differentiating acute fatty liver of pregnancy and HELLP syndrome is difficult, requiring liver biopsy as the gold standard. Delivery is the mainstay of treatment, because liver enzyme concentrations normalize shortly afterward.

SUPERIMPOSED PREECLAMPSIA

When pregnant women with chronic hypertension develop preeclampsia, it is known as superimposed preeclampsia. This condition is defined as a systolic BP greater than 140 mm Hg and a diastolic BP greater than 90 mm Hg, with evidence of preeclampsia (**Table 7**). It occurs in 8.7% to 25% of pregnant women.[9,11,12,32,61] Risk factors include antihypertensive use and African American ethnicity,[9] with conflicting data on body mass index.[9,32]

Table 7 Evidence of superimposed preeclampsia	
New-onset proteinuria >300 g/24 h	>2+ proteinuria on microanalysis
Sudden increase in proteinuria	Sudden increase in uncontrolled blood pressure
Platelets <100	Abnormal liver function tests >2× normal

Data from Samuel A, Lin C, Parviainen K, et al. Expectant management of preeclampsia superimposed on chronic hypertension. J Matern Fetal Neonatal Med 2011;24:907–11.

Superimposed preeclampsia results in maternal and perinatal morbidity and mortality, with increasing rates of pulmonary edema, postpartum hemorrhage, placental abruption,[12,61] and cesarean section.[61] There is also an increase in small for gestational age,[9] preterm delivery,[12] and neonatal mortality.[12] Assessment, diagnosis, and treatment are similar to those for patients with preeclampsia.

SUMMARY

Hypertensive disorders of pregnancy are becoming more prevalent. It is important for emergency medicine physicians to identify hypertensive pregnant women early. In this population, screening for end-organ damage, preeclampsia, eclampsia, HELLP syndrome, and fatty liver of pregnancy is best done early. Pregnant women with mild hypertension and no end-organ damage do not require any medication; however, those with BP higher than 150/100 mm Hg or end-organ damage require BP control. In severe cases, parenteral antihypertensive medications may be required. Emergency physicians should choose antihypertensive medications that they are comfortable using and that are safe in pregnancy. In women with preeclampsia, magnesium can prevent progression to eclampsia and is the medication of choice for eclamptic seizures. The definitive treatment for gestational hypertension, preeclampsia, eclampsia, HELLP syndrome, and fatty liver of pregnancy is delivery.

REFERENCES

1. Report of the national high blood pressure education program working group on high blood pressure in pregnancy. Am J Obstet Gynecol 2000;183:S1–22.
2. Steegers EA, von Dadelszen P, Duvekot JJ, et al. Pre-eclampsia. Lancet 2010; 376:631–44.
3. American College of Obstetricians and Gynecologists. Chronic hypertension in pregnancy. ACOG practice bulletin no. 125. Obstet Gynecol 2012;119:396–407.
4. Sibai BM. Chronic hypertension in pregnancy. Obstet Gynecol 2002;100:369–77.
5. Bateman BT, Bansil P, Hernandez-Diaz S, et al. Prevalence, trends, and outcomes of chronic hypertension: a nationwide sample of delivery admission. Am J Obstet Gynecol 2012;206:134.e1–8.
6. Magee LA, Abalos E, Dadelszen P, et al. How to manage hypertension in pregnancy effectively. Br J Clin Pharmacol 2011;72(3):394–401.
7. Sibai BM. Caring for women with hypertension in pregnancy. JAMA 2007;298: 1566–8.
8. Catov JM, Nohr EA, Olsen J, et al. Chronic hypertension related to risk for preterm and term small for gestational age births. Obstet Gynecol 2008;122:290–6.
9. Chappell L, Enye S, Paul S, et al. Adverse perinatal outcomes and risk factors for preeclampsia in women with chronic hypertension. Hypertension 2008;51: 1002–9.
10. James AH, Bushnell CD, Jamison MG, et al. Incidence and risk factors for stroke in pregnancy and the puerperium. Obstet Gynecol 2005;106:509–16.
11. Lindheimer M, Taler S, Cunningham F. Hypertension in pregnancy. J Am Soc Hypertens 2010;4:68–78.
12. Sibai BM, Lindheimer M, Hauth J, et al. Risk factors for preeclampsia, abruptio placentae, and adverse neonatal outcomes among women with chronic hypertension. N Engl J Med 1998;339:667–71.
13. Abalos E, Duley L, Steyn DW, et al. Antihypertensive drug therapy for mild to moderate hypertension during pregnancy. Cochrane Database Syst Rev 2007;1:CD002252.

14. von Dadelszen P, Ornstein M, Bull S, et al. Fall in mean arterial pressure and fetal growth restriction in pregnancy hypertension: a meta-analysis. Lancet 2000;355: 87–92.
15. Podymow T, August P. Antihypertensive drugs in pregnancy. Semin Nephrol 2011;31:70–85.
16. Kuklina EV, Tong X, Bansil P, et al. Trends in pregnancy hospitalizations that included a stroke in the United States from 1994 to 2007. Stroke 2011;42: 2564–70.
17. Martin J, Thigpen B, Moore R, et al. Stroke and severe preeclampsia and eclampsia: a paradigm shift focusing on systolic blood pressure. Obstet Gynecol 2005;105:246–54.
18. Chobanian A, Bakris G, Black H, et al. Joint National Committee on Prevention, Detection, Evaluation, and Treatment of High Blood Pressure; National Heart, Lung, and Blood Institute; National High Blood Pressure Education Program Coordinating Committee. Seventh report of the Joint National Committee on Prevention, Detection, Evaluation, and Treatment of High Blood Pressure. JAMA 2003;289:2560–71.
19. National Institute for Health and Clinical Excellence. Hypertension in pregnancy: the management of hypertensive disorders during pregnancy. NICE Clinical Guideline 107. London: NICE; 2010.
20. Powrie RA. 30-year-old woman with chronic hypertension trying to conceive. JAMA 2007;298:1548–99.
21. Duley L, Henderson-Smart DJ, Meher S. Drugs for treatment of very high blood pressure during pregnancy. Cochrane Database Syst Rev 2006;3:CD001449.
22. Cockburn J, Moar V, Ounsted M, et al. Final report of study on hypertension during pregnancy: the effects of specific treatment on the growth and development of the children. Lancet 1982;1:647–9.
23. Committee on Obstetric Practice. Committee opinion no. 514. Emergent therapy for acute-onset, severe hypertension with preeclampsia or eclampsia. Obstet Gynecol 2011;118:1465–8.
24. Cooper W, Hernandez-Diaz S, Arbogast P, et al. Major congenital malformations after first-trimester exposure to ACE inhibitors. N Engl J Med 2006;354:2443–51.
25. Villar J, Carroli G, Wojdyla D, et al. Preeclampsia, gestational hypertension and intrauterine growth restriction, related or independent conditions? Am J Obstet Gynecol 2006;194:921–31.
26. Weiss J, Malone F, Emig D, et al. Obesity, obstetric complications and cesarean delivery rate: a population based screening study. Am J Obstet Gynecol 2004; 190:1091–7.
27. Buchbinder A, Sabai BM, Caritis S, et al. Adverse perinatal outcomes are significantly higher in severe gestational hypertension than in mild preeclampsia. Am J Obstet Gynecol 2002;186:66–71.
28. Habli M, Levine RJ, Qian C, et al. Neonatal outcomes in pregnancies with preeclampsia or gestational hypertension and in normotensive pregnancies that delivered at 35, 36, or 37 weeks of gestation. Am J Obstet Gynecol 2007; 197:406.e1–7.
29. Sibai BM. Diagnosis and management of gestational hypertension and preeclampsia. Obstet Gynecol 2003;102:181–92.
30. Nabhan AF, Elsedawy MM. Tight control of mild-moderate pre-existing or non-proteinuric gestational hypertension. Cochrane Database Syst Rev 2011;7: CD006907.
31. Koopmans C, Bijlenga D, Groen H, et al. Induction of labour versus expectant monitoring for gestational hypertension or mild pre-eclampsia after 36 weeks'

gestation (HYPITAT): a multicentre, open-label randomised controlled trial. Lancet 2009;374:979–88.

32. Sibai BM. Management of late preterm and early-term pregnancies complicated by mild gestational hypertension/pre-eclampsia. Semin Perinatol 2011; 35:292–6.

33. Cote AM, Firoz T, Mattman A, et al. The 24-hour urine collection: gold standard or historical practice? Am J Obstet Gynecol 2008;199:625.e6.

34. Leeman L, Fontaine P. Hypertensive disorders of pregnancy. Am Fam Physician 2008;78:93–100.

35. Al-Safi Z, Imudia A, Filetti L, et al. Delayed postpartum preeclampsia and eclampsia. Obstet Gynecol 2011;118:1102–7.

36. Sibai BM, Koch MA, Freire S, et al. The impact of prior preeclampsia on the risk of superimposed preeclampsia and other adverse pregnancy outcomes in patients with chronic hypertension. Am J Obstet Gynecol 2011;204:345.e1–6.

37. Clarke S, Nelson-Piercy C. Pre-eclampsia and HELLP syndrome. Anaesth Intensive Care Med 2008;9:110–4.

38. Dekker G, Sibai B. Primary, secondary, and tertiary prevention of pre-eclampsia. Lancet 2001;357:209–15.

39. Caritis S, Sibai B, Hauth J, et al. Predictors of pre-eclampsia in women at high risk. Am J Obstet Gynecol 1998;179:946–51.

40. Ananth C, Savitz D, Williams M. Placental abruption and its association with hypertension and prolonged rupture of membranes: a methodological review and meta-analysis. Obstet Gynecol 1996;88:309–18.

41. Duley L, Henderson-Smart D, Meher S, et al. Antiplatelet agents for preventing pre-eclampsia and its complications. Cochrane Database Syst Rev 2007;2:CD004659.

42. Coomarasamy A, Honest H, Papioannou S, et al. Aspirin for prevention of preeclampsia in women with historical risk factors: a systematic review. Obstet Gynecol 2003;101:1319–32.

43. ACOG Committee on Obstetric Practice. Diagnosis and management of preeclampsia and eclampsia. ACOG practice bulletin no. 33. American College of Obstetricians and Gynecologists. Obstet Gynecol 2002;99:159–67.

44. Rumbold A, Duley L, Crowther CA, et al. Antioxidants for preventing pre-eclampsia. Cochrane Database Syst Rev 2008;1:CD004227.

45. Publications Committee, Society for Maternal-Fetal Medicine, Sibai B. Evaluation and management of severe preeclampsia before 34 weeks' gestation. Am J Obstet Gynecol 2011;205:191–8.

46. Duley L, Gülmezoglu AM, Henderson-Smart DJ, et al. Magnesium sulphate and other anticonvulsants for women with pre-eclampsia. Cochrane Database Syst Rev 2010;11:CD000025.

47. Duley L, Henderson-Smart DJ, Walker GJA, et al. Magnesium sulphate versus diazepam for eclampsia. Cochrane Database Syst Rev 2010;12:CD000127.

48. Duley L, Hendersone-Smart DJ, Chou D. Magnesium sulphate versus phenytoin for eclampsia. Cochrane Database Syst Rev 2010;10:CD000128.

49. Darngawn L, Jose R, Regi A, et al. A shortened postpartum magnesium sulfate prophylaxis regime in pre-eclamptic women at low risk of eclampsia. Int J Gynaecol Obstet 2012;116:237–9.

50. Ehrenberg H, Mercer B. Abbreviated postpartum magnesium sulfate therapy for women with mild preeclampsia. Obstet Gynecol 2006;108:833–8.

51. von Dadelszen P, Menzies J, Payne B, et al. Predicting adverse outcomes in women with severe pre-eclampsia. Semin Perinatol 2009;33:152–7.

52. Payne B, Magee L, von Dadelszen P. Assessment, surveillance and prognosis in pre-eclampsia. Best Pract Res Clin Obstet Gynaecol 2011;25:449–62.
53. von Dadelszen P, Payne B, Jing L, et al. Prediction of adverse maternal outcomes in pre-eclampsia: development and validation of the fullPIERS model. Lancet 2011;377:219–27.
54. Urato A, Bond B, Craigo S, et al. Admission uric acid levels and length of expectant management in preterm preeclampsia. J Perinatol 2011. [Epub ahead of print]. http://dx.doi.org/10.1038/jp.2011.187.
55. Belghiti J, Kayem G, Tsatsaris V, et al. Benefits and risks of expectant management of severe preeclampsia at less than 26 weeks gestation: the impact of gestational age and severe fetal growth restriction. Am J Obstet Gynecol 2011; 205:465.e1–6.
56. Bombrys AE, Barton JR, Nowacki EA, et al. Expectant management of severe preeclampsia at less than 27 weeks' gestation: maternal and perinatal outcomes according to gestational age by weeks at onset of expectant management. Am J Obstet Gynecol 2008;199:247.e1–6.
57. Morikawa M, Cho K, Yamada T, et al. Risk factors for eclampsia in Japan between 2005 and 2009. Int J Gynaecol Obstet 2012;117:66–8.
58. Liu S, Joseph KS, Liston RM, et al. Incidence, risk factors, and associated complications of eclampsia. Obstet Gynecol 2011;118:987–94.
59. Habli M, Eftekhari N, Wiebracht E, et al. Long-term maternal and subsequent pregnancy outcomes 5 years after hemolysis, elevated liver enzymes, and low platelets (HELLP) syndrome. Am J Obstet Gynecol 2009;201:385.e1–5.
60. Woudstra DM, Chandra S, Hofmeyr GJ, et al. Corticosteroids for HELLP (hemolysis, elevated liver enzymes, low platelets) syndrome in pregnancy. Cochrane Database Syst Rev 2010;9:CD008148.
61. Samuel A, Lin C, Parviainen K, et al. Expectant management of preeclampsia superimposed on chronic hypertension. J Matern Fetal Neonatal Med 2011;24: 907–11.

Complications in Late Pregnancy

David Meguerdichian, MD[a,b,*]

KEYWORDS

- Late pregnancy • Placenta previa • Abruptio placenta • Amniotic fluid embolus
- Preterm pregnancy • Braxton Hicks contractions
- Preterm premature rupture of membranes • Uterine rupture

KEY POINTS

- Managing complications of late pregnancy requires prompt maternal and fetal evaluation as well as an understanding of hospital protocols so patients can have appropriate triage and treatment.
- Abruptio placentae classically presents as painful, third-trimester bleeding in contrast to the often painless bleeding of placenta previa.
- Ultrasound imaging is most useful in ruling out placenta previa and should not delay care in unstable third-trimester bleeding patients.
- In the intrapartum or early postpartum period, evidence of hypotension, respiratory distress, or disseminated intravascular coagulation suggests amniotic fluid embolism and requires aggressive resuscitative measures.
- Corticosteroid administration is the most beneficial antenatal intervention in preterm labor.
- Uterine rupture should be suspected in patients with a history of uterine surgery who present with abdominal pain, vaginal bleeding, and cessation of uterine contractions.
- Appropriate management of late pregnancy complications requires prompt treatment of hemodynamic instability, evaluation of maternal and fetal welfare, and early obstetric consultation.

INTRODUCTION

Complications of late pregnancy are seen with less frequency in the emergency department (ED) than those of the first trimester (eg, spontaneous abortion and ectopic pregnancy). In many hospitals, the lower frequency is the result of an institutional policy that triages many of these patients directly to the labor and delivery unit. Nonetheless, emergency medicine (EM) physicians must be comfortable in identifying

There is no funding support for this article. The author has nothing to disclose.
[a] Harvard Medical School, 25 Shattuck Street, Boston, MA 02115, USA; [b] Department of Emergency Medicine, Brigham and Women's Hospital, 75 Francis Street, Neville House, Boston, MA 02115, USA
* Department of Emergency Medicine, Brigham and Women's Hospital, 75 Francis Street, Neville House, Boston, MA 02115.
E-mail address: dmeguerdichian@partners.org

Emerg Med Clin N Am 30 (2012) 919–936
http://dx.doi.org/10.1016/j.emc.2012.08.002
0733-8627/12/$ – see front matter © 2012 Elsevier Inc. All rights reserved.

emed.theclinics.com

and addressing these complications, given the profound impact they can have on maternal and fetal health. The emergencies of late pregnancy include abruptio placentae, placenta previa, amniotic fluid embolism, preterm labor, preterm premature rupture of membranes, and uterine rupture. This article discusses the clinical presentations, the risk factors, and the most current diagnostic approaches and management strategies for the key complications that EM physicians will encounter in late-pregnancy patients.

ABRUPTIO PLACENTAE
Causes and Risk Factors

Abruptio placentae is the separation of an implanted placenta after the twentieth week of pregnancy and before actual delivery.[1,2] The separation can be complete or partial, with bleeding into the decidua basalis.[1] Bleeding can remain concealed and undetected or track between the membranes, subsequently escaping through the cervix.[3] This hemorrhage causes compression of the intervillous space and ultimately placental tissue damage.[2] Mechanisms for abruption seem to be multifactorial and include impaired placentation, poor perfusion/hypoxia to the uteroplacental interface, and placental insufficiency.[4,5] The symptoms of abruption range from none to severe hemorrhage with subsequent fetal death and maternal morbidity, making this diagnosis challenging for the EM physician. Risk factors associated with abruptio placentae are listed in **Box 1**.[2,6]

Clinical Presentation

The most common presenting symptoms of placental abruption are vaginal bleeding, uterine contractions, abdominal pain, and uterine tenderness.[4] Vaginal bleeding occurs in 80% of cases; the blood is usually dark, and the amount correlates poorly with the degree of abruption.[1] Other symptoms may include back pain, nausea, vomiting, and reduced fetal movements. The maternal coagulation cascade can be activated at any time during this process and result in disseminated intravascular coagulation (DIC).[7] In severe abruptio placentae, the uterus becomes severely contracted and painful, maternal hypotension ensues, and fetal death is possible.[2]

Box 1
Risk factors associated with abruptio placentae

- History of abruptio placentae
- Maternal hypertensive disease (preeclampsia, chronic hypertension)
- Cigarette smoking
- Cocaine/vasoconstrictive drug use
- Abdominal trauma
- Multiple pregnancies
- Chorioamnionitis
- Placental abnormalities
- Folate deficiencies
- Premature rupture of membranes
- Hyperhomocysteinemia
- Thrombophilia

Cardiotocogram monitoring can demonstrate a variety of heart rhythms and contractions when abruptio placentae is present. Classically, the uterine contractions have a high-frequency, low-amplitude pattern with an elevated baseline tone. Fetal heart rates can show recurrent late or variable decelerations, bradycardia, or sinusoidal patterns.[2,7]

Classification

Abruptio placentae has been categorized into 3 grades that describe the clinical findings[1,8]:

- Grade 1 (40% of cases): slight vaginal bleeding, uterine irritability, no maternal distress, no fetal distress
- Grade 2 (45% of cases): mild to moderate vaginal bleeding, uterine contractions, little maternal distress, presence of fetal distress
- Grade 3 (15% of cases): severe vaginal bleeding; painful, tetanic uterus; maternal hypotension and coagulopathy; fetal distress and, often, death

Diagnosis

Clinical

The diagnosis of abruptio placentae is a clinical one and should be considered in any late-pregnancy patient presenting to the ED with vaginal bleeding, abdominal pain, recent trauma, or signs of preterm labor. In moderate to severe cases, the diagnosis is often clear and made before delivery; in mild cases, the diagnosis is delayed until after delivery and based on the evaluation of a retroplacental clot.[2] The main alternative diagnosis in women with late-pregnancy bleeding is placenta previa. The alternative considerations are clearly broader for late-pregnancy women who present with abdominal pain and include those listed below:

- Premature labor
- Complications of preeclampsia
- Hepatic and gallbladder disease
- Appendicitis
- Ovarian torsion

Ultrasound

Similar to its clinical presentation, abruptio placentae has a variety of ultrasonographic appearances. Factors, such as size of the bleed, location of the bleed, and duration between the abruption and time to evaluation, play a part in how well the abruption can be observed.[7,9] Small and acute bleeds are difficult to appreciate because they can be isoechoic in comparison with the placenta; larger, concealed bleeds are usually more easily visualized.[10] When a clot is identified on the ultrasound image, this finding has an 88% positive predictive value for abruption (**Fig. 1**).[10] Ultrasound is a tool for monitoring expectant cases and excluding placenta previa, but it should never be used to examine unstable patients because it can delay definitive care.[2]

Kleihauer-Betke test

The Kleihauer-Betke test is performed frequently but shows limited usefulness in the diagnosis of abruptio placentae. A retrospective cohort study using this test found no positive tests among placentas later identified as having undergone abruption on pathologic review.[11] Thus, this test cannot be used to confirm or rule out abruption. The Kleihauer-Betke test is better applied for quantifying fetomaternal transfusion to guide the administration of Rh-immune globulin to an Rh-negative mother.[7]

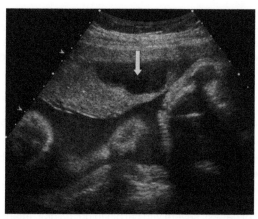

Fig. 1. Ultrasound image showing acute placental abruption with a retroplacental hematoma (*arrow*) lifting part of the placenta. (*Courtesy of* Carol Benson, MD, Brigham and Women's Hospital Department of Radiology.)

Treatment

The treatment strategies for abruptio placentae rely heavily on the presentation and state of the mother and fetus. Many institutions have protocols for triaging and evaluating obstetrics patients either in the ED or in the labor and delivery suite. The EM physician should use these protocols to guide initial management. If no obstetric services are available in the institution, the patient's own obstetrician should be involved promptly. When the diagnosis is uncertain and the presentation is mild, the treating physician can rely on expectant management. At the other end of the spectrum, severe abruptio placentae calls for immediate hemodynamic stabilization of the mother and delivery of the baby.[2] Overall, the care of abruptio placentae must be tailored on a case-by-case basis.

Stable mother and fetus

The initial evaluation of stable patients with abruption begins by placing them in a monitored bed and obtaining intravenous (IV) access with 2 large-bore catheters. If patients are at or near full term with imminent delivery, vaginal delivery is preferred if it can be tolerated by the mother and fetus. This delivery should occur in a setting capable of progressing to cesarean section. For mothers who are preterm and medically stable, expectant management is safe and appropriate.[12–14] In fact, a retrospective study of 131 patients with abruption demonstrated that tocolysis is safe for use in preterm abruptio placentae.[12] In all cases, the mother and fetus must be monitored and reevaluated continuously because a stable abruption can progress to an unstable abruption, causing patients to deteriorate rapidly.

Unstable mother or fetus

As with any unstable patient presenting to the ED, the initial management of patients with severe abruptio placentae involves placing them in a monitored bed, obtaining IV access with 2 large-bore catheters, and performing a primary survey. On their arrival in the ED, a complete blood count should be requested and a blood-bank specimen should be collected for type and crossmatch, coagulation studies, and Rh testing. Patients who are hypotensive should be treated initially with IV normal saline and transitioned to packed red blood cells if they are unresponsive to this initial intervention. Once the mother stabilizes, the fetus can be evaluated with ultrasound imaging to rule out placenta previa and monitor the heart rate.[2] If the fetus is viable, delivery should be expedited in the operating room with a double setup for delivery. Vaginal delivery is acceptable until fetal monitoring shows signs of distress or maternal surveillance shows evidence of deterioration.[2,7] At this point, cesarean delivery should be performed because complete placental detachment is imminent and could occur at any time.[7] Meticulous monitoring should be performed at all times for signs of hemorrhagic shock and DIC, which are 2 complications commonly associated with abruptio placentae. Hemorrhagic shock should be addressed with transfusion aimed at restoring appropriate circulating blood volume. DIC is more commonly seen after fetal death, and its management involves treating the underlying condition with delivery of the fetus and placenta.[2,15] Vaginal delivery is the route of choice in such cases, but cesarean section might be indicated for maternal reasons and can be performed once DIC is reversed.[2,7] Resolution of coagulopathy is rapid following delivery but can be augmented with the addition of fresh frozen plasma (FFP).

Placental abruption continues to be a key cause of perinatal morbidity and mortality. Prompt recognition of this condition is vital for the well-being of the fetus and the mother. Expectant management is appropriate in preterm cases with a stable patient and fetus, whereas emergent delivery is key to management for mature term or unstable cases.

PLACENTA PREVIA
Causes and Risk Factors

Placenta previa is the implantation of the placenta overlying or within 2 cm of the internal cervical os.[16,17] In placenta previa, the placenta implants partially or fully in the lower uterine segment, as opposed to the upper uterine segment, as in normal pregnancy.[18] Placenta previa has been classified into 4 categories based on the placenta's location[18]:

- Complete: placenta completely covers the internal os
- Partial: placenta partially covers the internal os
- Marginal: placenta just reaches but does not cover the internal os
- Low lying: placenta extends into the lower uterine segment, with no approximation to the internal os

Placenta previa occurs in 0.3% to 0.5% of pregnancies.[19,20] The exact cause of implantation of the placenta in the lower uterine segment is unclear. Uterine scarring is one proposed predisposing factor.[18] In many cases, low-implanting placentas move away from the cervix and toward the better-vascularized fundus as the pregnancy progresses.[18] Factors that seem to increase the risk of placenta previa are listed in **Box 2**.[19,21]

Box 2
Risk factors for placenta previa
• Advanced maternal age
• Multiparity
• Cigarette smoking
• Previous cesarean sections
• Chronic hypertension
• Multiple gestations
• Uterine surgery

Clinical Presentation

Placenta previa is a common incidental finding seen in 4% of regular second-trimester ultrasound studies and only 0.4% by the time all pregnancies reach term.[19,21–23] In contrast to the usual painful presentation of abruptio placentae, symptomatic placenta previa is characterized by painless, bright-red vaginal bleeding at or after the end of the second trimester.[18] The initial sentinel bleed rarely causes hemodynamic instability unless the placenta is further disrupted by cervical instrumentation or digital examination, which can cause severe hemorrhage.[17] Despite being classified as painless, placenta previa bleeding can occur in women in active labor who are experiencing pain from contractions.

Diagnosis

Ultrasound is the diagnostic modality of choice for localizing and identifying placenta previa. Transvaginal ultrasonography is the most accurate means of visualizing 2 key structures, the placenta and cervical os, which are often obscured on the transabdominal approach by the fetus and the maternal bony pelvis.[22] In one study, crucial landmarks were identified poorly on 50% of transabdominal ultrasound images; this series also showed 26% fewer cases of placenta previa when a transvaginal approach was used in suspected cases.[24] This approach, when performed by properly trained personnel, is safe and does not lead to an increased risk of bleeding.[25,26]

Treatment

Placenta previa must be considered in all women in late pregnancy presenting to the ED with vaginal bleeding. The initial assessment includes maternal evaluation, with emphasis on identifying abnormal vital signs, performing a primary survey, and establishing IV access with 2 large-bore catheters. A complete blood count, type and crossmatch, Rh-status study, and coagulation studies should be requested. Continuous fetal monitoring should also be prioritized during this initial management period. An ultrasound study can be performed to locate the placenta and diagnose placenta previa.

If hypotension or severe hemorrhage is identified, the mother and fetus can be resuscitated initially with IV normal saline boluses and ultimately with crossmatched packed red blood cells, as for abruptio placentae. Once the mother is stabilized, she should be transferred to the obstetric unit for further management; if this resource is not available, she should be transferred, accompanied by a high-acuity transfer team, to an appropriate receiving hospital.

Following stabilization of the patient, the goal of the EM physician is to prolong pregnancy until the fetal lungs mature.[17] Under the guidance of an obstetrician, various strategies can be used to achieve this goal. Tocolytic agents safely prolong pregnancy in patients with vaginal bleeding and preterm contractions.[27] Administration of corticosteroids can be considered to promote lung maturation in the fetus of women who present with placenta previa bleeding at 24 to 34 weeks' gestation.[28,29] These patients should have a neonatology consultation to better understand the management of the child following premature birth.[18]

Cervical cerclage has been proposed as an intervention for prolonging pregnancy in patients with placenta previa. This intervention has shown mixed results; one small study showed improved outcomes, including mean birth weight and greater gestational age at delivery, whereas another small study showed no statistically significant difference between the outcomes in the cerclage group versus controls.[30,31] A

Cochrane meta-analysis demonstrated that cerclage may lessen the risk of delivery before 34 weeks, yet the investigators argued for further studies before recommending that this practice be made the standard of care.[32]

Following any or all of these interventions, patients should be admitted for close monitoring to allow fetal maturation and a safe, successful delivery. Women who are stable, asymptomatic, and reliable and who can rapidly return to labor and delivery can be managed as outpatients at the discretion of their obstetricians.[18]

AMNIOTIC FLUID EMBOLISM
Causes and Risk Factors

Amniotic fluid embolism (AFE) is a rare, catastrophic, and often fatal complication of late pregnancy. The pathogenesis and disease process remain poorly understood, even though AFE is one of the main causes of maternal mortality in the United States.[33] The pathogenesis of AFE is thought to be the introduction of amniotic fluid and debris into the systemic maternal circulation, with resultant physical obstruction in the pulmonary vasculature. However, autopsy studies and the inability to reproduce the disease in animal models have sparked other theories to explain the mechanism for this maternal complication.[34] Some investigators have proposed that the hemodynamic manifestation of AFE is comparable with that of anaphylactic shock and hypothesized that an immunologic mechanism drives the process.[35–38] More recently, complement activation has been proposed as playing a role in the pathogenesis of AFE, with more promising serologic and histologic evidence than prior hypotheses.[35,38,39] Despite the lack of a definitive understanding, it does seem more convincing that the introduction of amniotic fluid into the maternal circulation results in the release of several endogenous mediators that trigger the physiologic presentation of this disease.[34] Risk factors for AFE were elucidated in 2 recent retrospective studies **(Box 3)**.[40,41]

Clinical Presentation

AFE usually occurs intrapartum or during the initial postpartum period. The symptoms are typically sudden in onset and can occur as late as 48 hours after delivery.[34,42] The most common signs and symptoms of AFE are the following[34,43]:

- Hypotension
- Fetal distress
- Pulmonary edema/respiratory distress
- Cardiac arrest

Box 3
Risk factors for amniotic fluid embolism

- Maternal age more than 35 years
- Cesarean delivery
- Forceps or vacuum-assisted delivery
- Abruptio placentae
- Placenta previa
- Eclampsia
- Fetal distress

- Cyanosis
- Coagulopathy/DIC

Initially, patients experience the release of vasoactive substances, causing vaso-spasm, pulmonary hypertension, and subsequent cardiovascular collapse.[36,44] Survi-vors of this initial offense are usually confronted with the challenges of DIC, left ventricular dysfunction, and pulmonary edema.[36,44] Maternal death from AFE is typi-cally caused by acute cardiac arrest, severe hemorrhage from DIC, or the develop-ment of acute respiratory distress syndrome with subsequent multiorgan failure following survival of the initial event.[34]

Diagnosis

The diagnosis of AFE is based on the clinical presentation and should be suspected in women displaying hypotension, respiratory distress, or evidence of DIC during the intrapartum period or the first 48 hours after delivery.[34] The diagnosis is essentially made by excluding other medical conditions or explanations of patients' symptoms and is usually made with certainty only at autopsy.[34] Intravascular fetal material, tryp-tase, and complement can be elevated in patients with AFE.[34,35] These diagnostic markers could be promising, but further investigation is required. General laboratory and imaging studies are nonspecific but should be used by the EM physician to guide ED management of these critically ill patients. These studies include a complete blood count, coagulation studies, arterial blood gas measurements, cardiac markers, an electrocardiogram, a chest radiograph, and possible bedside echocardiography.

Treatment

Proper management of AFE requires early recognition and prompt initiation of neces-sary supportive and resuscitative measures. The initial treatment involves identifying abnormal vital signs, commencing cardiorespiratory monitoring, and rapidly perform-ing a primary survey.

Following the primary evaluation, treatment of AFE should focus on airway control, hemodynamic stability, and correction of coagulopathy.[42] Control of the airway from the onset is key because some form of hypoxia is present with AFE. Early tracheal intubation with 100% oxygen administration and positive-pressure ventilation should be achieved without delay. Two large-bore IV catheters should be placed to allow rapid resuscitation with normal saline and packed red blood cells if hypotension or severe bleeding ensues. Vasopressors, such as dopamine and norepinephrine, and inotropes, such as dobutamine and milrinone, can be used to address refractory hypotension, with a goal systolic blood pressure of greater than 90 mm Hg. Progres-sion to vasopressors should prompt central venous catheter placement, which also allows closer central pressure monitoring and sampling. Other blood products, such as FFP, platelets, and cryoprecipitate, should be available for administration if coagulopathy develops.[45] The EM physician's main goal, as with all cases of cardio-pulmonary collapse, should be rapid protection of the airway, correction of hemody-namic instability, and prompt admission to the intensive care unit for further monitoring and management.

FALSE LABOR/BRAXTON HICKS CONTRACTIONS

Braxton Hicks contractions, named after the physician who first described this phenomenon in 1872, are classified as irregular, uncoordinated, painful, or painless contractions, which can be easily confused with true labor.[46] After 30 weeks, the intensity of these contractions can increase and patients may describe a greater firmness in their lower abdomen. Contrary to true labor, these contractions are not associated with demonstrable cervical effacement and dilatation.[46]

Diagnosis

False labor is usually a clinical diagnosis. Examination of the cervix, with care to not disrupt the intact membrane, will show minimal dilation.[47] External tocometric monitoring can be performed and will show no increase in the frequency or duration of the uterine contractions, as is seen in true labor.[47]

Treatment

Braxton Hicks contractions are typically managed with hydration, bed rest, and analgesia as needed. An obstetrician can be consulted when the distinction between true and false labor remains unclear.

PRETERM LABOR
Causes and Risk Factors

Preterm labor (PTL) is defined by the World Health Organization as the onset of delivery at or before 37 weeks' gestation.[48,49] Preterm delivery occurs in roughly 12% of all live births in the United States and remains a major cause of perinatal morbidity and mortality.[50,51] Because of the often-unexpected nature of PTL, the EM physician should be comfortable in evaluating and managing patients with this condition in the ED.

The causes of PTL are multifactorial and closely tied to several clinical factors[49,52]:

- Psychosocial factors
  - Low socioeconomic status
  - Extremes of age (<18 or >40 years)
  - Tobacco use
  - Substance abuse (cocaine)
  - Nonwhite race
- Maternal reproductive and gynecologic factors
  - History of preterm labor
  - Low pregnancy weight
  - Prior second-trimester abortion
  - Multiple gestations
  - Uterine anomalies
  - Cervical incompetence
  - History of placental abruption or previa
- Infections of the genital and urinary tract

Clinical Presentation

Understanding and identifying the signs and symptoms of PTL will allow the EM physician to diagnose and treat this condition expeditiously. Typical presentations include uterine activity with frequent contractions of more than 4 per hour, cramping abdominal pain, pelvic pressure, an increase or change in vaginal discharge, back pain, and vaginal bleeding.[52,53]

Diagnosis

PTL can be diagnosed on clinical grounds when patients are between 20 and 36 weeks' gestation and demonstrates the following[48]:

- Painful contractions lasting longer than 30 seconds and occurring at least 4 times every 20 minutes

- A change in the position, length, or dilation of the cervix, usually with effacement of at least 80% and dilation greater than 2 cm

Useful ED studies include a complete blood count, urinalysis, and pelvic ultrasonography. Emergent ultrasonography, which has been shown to be far superior to the vaginal digital examination, can allow assessment for cervical shortening—a finding that places patients at a higher risk for preterm delivery.[54–56] Aside from assessing cervical length, ultrasound examination can identify fetal anomalies, fetal presentation, placenta previa, abruptio placentae, or fetal demise, giving the obstetrics team information that can be used to counsel patients on expected outcomes.[57] A growing body of obstetrics literature is showing that the finding of fetal fibronectin in cervical or vaginal fluid augments imaging in identifying patients at risk for PTL.[58–60] All of the aforementioned studies can be done in the ED or labor and delivery, depending on hospital protocols and urgency of delivery.

Treatment

In the presence of a viable fetus and healthy mother, the management of preterm labor relies on several medical modalities. The hallmarks of management are the use of tocolytics to prolong pregnancy and the administration of medications to promote fetal maturity.

Tocolytic therapy

The primary aim of tocolytic therapy is to arrest premature labor and imminent delivery for up to 48 hours.[61] Tocolytic medications should be administered in the ED in consultation with an obstetrician. Ultimately, a delay in delivery is sought to allow increased time for 2 key steps[48,52,61]:

- Administration of a complete course of antenatal glucocorticosteroids aimed at promoting fetal lung maturity
- Transfer to a tertiary obstetrics and pediatric center or unit that is capable of managing preterm labor and a premature infant

Several contraindications to tocolysis exist and should be considered before initiating therapy[52]:

- Fetal distress
- Preeclampsia or eclampsia
- Fetal demise
- Chorioamnionitis
- DIC
- Acute vaginal bleeding
- Preterm premature rupture of membranes

Evidence supports the use of β-adrenergic receptor agonists, calcium channel blockers, magnesium sulfate, and nonsteroidal antiinflammatory drugs (NSAIDs) as first-line agents for tocolysis.[61] A recent meta-analysis showed benefit of these agents versus placebo alone for delaying delivery but also showed that NSAIDs might be the superior first-line agent because of their tolerability and fewer maternal/fetal side effects.[62] The side-effect profiles of each agent (**Box 4**) should be reviewed and discussed with the consulting obstetrician before initiating therapy.[52,61]

Titratable IV tocolytics should be administered first, while coordinating transfer to a labor and delivery unit, to identify the dose necessary for uterine contraction cessation. It is critical that every patient undergoing tocolytic therapy have external fetal heart monitoring to ensure prompt identification of fetal distress.

Box 4
Side effects of tocolytic agents

- β-Adrenergic drugs (terbutaline, ritodrine)
  - Pulmonary edema
  - Tachycardia
  - Hypokalemia
  - Hyperglycemia
- NSAIDs (indomethacin, ketorolac)
  - Prolonged bleeding
  - Gastrointestinal disturbance/bleeding
  - Fetal patent ductus arteriosus constriction
  - Fetal necrotizing enterocolitis
- Magnesium sulfate
  - Respiratory depression
  - Cardiac arrest
  - Loss of deep tendon reflexes
- Calcium channel blockers (nifedipine)
  - Hypotension
  - Bradycardia
  - Dizziness

Corticosteroid therapy

Antenatal corticosteroid administration is the most beneficial intervention for improved neonatal outcomes in patients who deliver preterm.[48,52,61] This intervention is beneficial regardless of the maternal membrane status. Its use results in lower severity and frequency of respiratory distress syndrome, intracranial hemorrhage, necrotizing enterocolitis, and death compared with those not receiving therapy.[29] The most commonly used and studied corticosteroids are betamethasone and dexamethasone, administered via either of the 2 regimens listed here[63]:

- Two 12-mg doses of betamethasone given intramuscularly 24 hours apart
- Four 6-mg doses of dexamethasone given intramuscularly every 12 hours

Antibiotics

Several maternal infections have been implicated as having a role in preterm labor, specifically at less than 32 weeks.[61] Treatment with antibiotics has shown no benefit in prolonging pregnancy or avoiding preterm delivery.[61] Nonetheless, women should be treated for sexually transmitted, urinary tract, respiratory, and vaginal infections if they are identified on testing. Group B streptococci screening should be performed, and positive or high-risk mothers should be treated with penicillin G (5 million units IV followed by 2.5 million units every 4 hours until delivery) to prevent vertical transmission of this infection to the newborn. In cases of preterm labor with rupture of membranes, a 48-hour course of ampicillin and erythromycin, followed by 5 days of amoxicillin and erythromycin, should be used to prolong pregnancy and reduce the risk of neonatal morbidity from infection transmission.[64]

PRETERM PREMATURE RUPTURE OF MEMBRANES
Causes and Risk Factors

Premature rupture of membranes (PROM) is the rupture of the amniotic membrane before the onset of labor. This outcome is classified as preterm PROM (PPROM) if it occurs before 37 weeks' gestation. PROM complicates close to 8% of pregnancies.[60,64] At term, normal weakening of the membranes is caused by physiologic changes and the force of uterine contractions.[65] The weakening seen with PROM has been associated with the risk factors listed in **Box 5**.[64,66,67] However, PROM can occur even in patients with none of the identified risk factors.

Diagnosis

Rupture of membranes typically presents as a large release of clear vaginal fluid or a regular trickle. From the outset, PROM can be diagnosed with an accurate history and physical examination. Special care must be taken with the physical examination to avoid the introduction of infection. A digital cervical examination should be avoided in particular because it provides little information over a speculum examination and raises the risk of infection or rupture of intact membranes.[64] With a sterile speculum examination, the ED physician can diagnose membrane rupture by visualizing the passage of fluid from the cervix. If in doubt, the additional diagnostic strategies listed here can be used[64]:

- pH measurement (Amniotic fluid has a basic pH of 7.1–7.3 compared with the more acidic vaginal secretions.)
- Applying posterior fornix fluid to a microscope slide and observing ferning under a microscope

Management

The initial evaluation of patients presenting to the ED with PROM requires an accurate determination of gestational age, an assessment of maternal/fetal risk factors, and prompt evaluation and counseling of patients in concert with their obstetrician. If gestational age is uncertain from the menstrual history or previous imaging, an ED ultrasound study can be performed to provide an estimate of gestational age. All patients with PROM should be evaluated for infection in similar fashion to patients

---

Box 5
Risk factors for PROM

- Intra-amniotic infection
- Poor socioeconomic status
- Late pregnancy bleeding
- Low body mass index
- Tobacco use
- Amniocentesis
- Copper and ascorbic acid nutritional deficiencies
- Connective tissue disorders
- Previous preterm birth
- Short cervical length

in preterm labor. The incidence of infection in PROM increases with decreased gestational age; 13% to 60% of patients with PPROM have clinically evident intra-amniotic infection.[64] Testing for *Chlamydia*, *Neisseria gonorrhoeae*, urinary tract infections, and group B streptococci should be requested and, if present, treated to avoid the onset of overt infectious symptoms and to prevent vertical transmission to the fetus. Electronic fetal heart rate monitoring should be initiated to assess for occult umbilical cord compression and fetal distress.

Term patients with PROM generally experience the prompt onset of labor and delivery. Oxytocin induction can be considered to decrease the period between PROM and delivery as well as the frequency of chorioamnionitis.[68] Patients with PPROM, similar to PTL management, require transfer or admission to an obstetrics unit to initiate preterm treatments, including the following:

- Antenatal glucocorticoid therapy to promote fetal lung maturity
- Tocolytic drugs to delay delivery for up to 48 hours to allow maximum effect of the glucocorticoids
- A 48-hour course of IV ampicillin and erythromycin followed by 5 days of amoxicillin and erythromycin to prolong pregnancy and decrease infection in cases remote from term
- Chemoprophylaxis to prevent vertical transmission of group B streptococci

Unlike some cases of PTL, women with PROM and PPROM cannot be managed with home care because of the usual brevity of the latent period, the rapidity with which fetal infection may occur, and the need for close fetal monitoring.[64]

UTERINE RUPTURE
Causes and Risk Factors

Rupture of the gravid uterus is a rare, life-threatening complication for both the mother and fetus. It is defined as direct communication between the uterine and peritoneal spaces following disruption of the uterine wall.[69] Uterine ruptures can be classified as either partial or complete and by their cause[70]:

- Traumatic
  - Obstetric (forceps use, fundal pressure)
  - Nonobstetric (violence, car crashes)
- Spontaneous
  - Previous uterine surgery
  - Unscarred uterus

The main risk factor for uterine rupture is a scarred uterus, which is usually secondary to a previous cesarean section.[70–72] A fair amount of recent literature focuses on uterine rupture as a result of women attempting vaginal birth after previous cesarean delivery.[70] Risk factors are listed in **Box 6**.[72]

Clinical Presentation

Maternal manifestations of uterine rupture usually include the acute onset of abdominal pain, cessation of uterine contractions, and various degrees of vaginal bleeding.[70,73] As in any severe intra-abdominal catastrophe, the patient can shows signs of shock, including hypotension and tachycardia. Fetal manifestations of uterine rupture include bradycardia, variable or late decelerations, and fetal demise.[70,74]

Box 6
Risk factors for uterine rupture

- Previous cesarean delivery
- Uterine surgery
- Congenital uterine malformations/abnormal uterine anatomy
- Labor-induction agents
- Trauma
- Elective abortion
- Advance maternal age
- Multiple gestations
- Abnormal placentation

Diagnosis

The diagnosis of uterine rupture can be challenging. A history of uterine surgery should place this diagnosis high on the differential for the EM physician treating symptomatic second- or third-trimester gravid patients. Uterine rupture is quite rare among women with unscarred uteri. As with any patient with abdominal pain and possible shock, basic laboratory studies, such as a complete blood count, coagulation studies, and a type and crossmatch for blood products, should be performed. Imaging studies, such as ultrasonography, might identify a uterine wall defect, a fetal anatomy protruding from the uterus, or signs of free fluid in the pelvis, which will help the EM physician care for these critically ill patients.[75]

Management

On initial presentation, patients with suspected uterine rupture should be placed in a monitored bed, have 2 large-bore IV catheters inserted for access, and undergo a primary survey, with attention to abnormal vital signs and evidence of shock. Patients who are hypotensive and those with evidence of severe hemorrhage should be stabilized with IV normal saline boluses and ultimately with crossmatched packed red blood cells, if indicated. Once the mother is safely stabilized, she should be transferred expeditiously to the obstetric unit or operating room for cesarean delivery. Early transfer and involvement of an obstetrician is key because it allows maximal fetal outcome and repair of the injured uterus. Smaller ruptures can undergo primary repair; women with large ruptures and those complicated by severe hemorrhage should undergo hysterectomy.[76] Future hopes of childbearing are taken into consideration, but the mother's condition and the extent of the injury usually dictate whether she should undergo repair or definitive hysterectomy.

SUMMARY

Complications of late pregnancy are managed infrequently in the ED and, thus, can pose a challenge when encountered as an acute presentation by the EM physician. Emergency care of these conditions requires rapid assessment, identification of hemodynamically unstable patients, and prompt intervention. Care must be taken to evaluate and manage both maternal and fetal well-being. Aside from addressing hemodynamic instability, focused care should include strategies to promote fetal maturity and prevent vertical transmission of infection if delivery is imminent. Early obstetrics consultation and involvement, as well as an understanding of one's own hospital triaging policies for third-trimester pregnancy, will allow appropriate and timely disposition plans for these patients.

REFERENCES

1. Tikkanen M. Etiology, clinical manifestations, and prediction of placental abruption. Acta Obstet Gynecol Scand 2010;89:732–40.
2. Hall DR. Abruptio placentae and disseminated intravascular coagulopathy. Semin Perinatol 2009;33:189–95.
3. Baron F, Hill WC. Placenta previa, placenta abruptio. Clin Obstet Gynecol 1998; 41:527–32.
4. Tikkanen M, Nuutila M, Hiilesmaa V, et al. Clinical presentation and risk factors of placental abruption. Acta Obstet Gynecol Scand 2006;85:700–5.
5. Kramer MS, Usher RH, Pollack R, et al. Etiologic determinants of abruptio placentae. Obstet Gynecol 1997;89:221–6.
6. Tikkanen M. Placental abruption: epidemiology, risk factors and consequences. Acta Obstet Gynecol Scand 2011;90:140–9.
7. Oyelese Y, Ananth CV. Placental abruption. Obstet Gynecol 2006;108:1005–16.
8. Hurd WW, Miodovnik M, Hertzberg V, et al. Selective management of abruptio placentae: a prospective study. Obstet Gynecol 1983;61:467–73.
9. Nyberg DA, Cyr DR, Mack LA, et al. Sonographic spectrum of placental abruption. AJR Am J Roentgenol 1987;148:161–4.
10. Glantz C, Purnell L. Clinical utility of sonography in the diagnosis and treatment of placental abruption. J Ultrasound Med 2002;21:837–40.
11. Emery CL, Morway LF, Chung-Park M, et al. The Kleihauer-Betke test: clinical utility, indication, and correlation in patients with placental abruption and cocaine use. Arch Pathol Lab Med 1995;119:1032–7.
12. Towers CV, Pircon RA, Heppard M. Is tocolysis safe in the management of third-trimester bleeding? Am J Obstet Gynecol 1999;180:1572–8.
13. Saller DN Jr, Nagey DA, Pupkin MJ, et al. Tocolysis in the management of third trimester bleeding. J Perinatol 1990;10:125–8.
14. Combs CA, Nyberg DA, Mack LA, et al. Expectant management after sonographic diagnosis of placental abruption. Am J Perinatol 1992;9:170–4.
15. Su LL, Chong YS. Massive obstetric haemorrhage with disseminated intravascular coagulopathy. Best Pract Res Clin Obstet Gynaecol 2012;26:77–90.
16. Bhide A, Prefumo F, Moore J, et al. Placental edge to internal os distance in the late third trimester and mode of delivery in placenta praevia. BJOG 2003;110: 860–4.
17. Sakornbut E, Leeman L, Fontaine P. Late pregnancy bleeding. Am Fam Physician 2007;75:1199–206.
18. Oyelese Y, Smulian JC. Placenta previa, placenta accreta, and vasa previa. Obstet Gynecol 2006;107:927–91.
19. Rosenberg T, Pariente G, Sergienko R, et al. Critical analysis of risk factors and outcome of placenta previa. Arch Gynecol Obstet 2011;284:47–51.
20. Iyasu S, Saftlas AK, Rowley DL, et al. The epidemiology of placenta previa in the United States, 1979 through 1987. Am J Obstet Gynecol 1993;168:1424–9.
21. Faiz AS, Ananth CV. Etiology and risk factors for placenta previa: an overview and meta-analysis of observational studies. J Matern Fetal Neonatal Med 2003;13: 175–90.

22. Mustafa SA, Brizot ML, Carvalho MH, et al. Transvaginal ultrasonography in predicting placenta previa at delivery: a longitudinal study. Ultrasound Obstet Gynecol 2002;20:356–9.
23. Bhide A, Thilaganathan B. Recent advances in the management of placenta previa. Curr Opin Obstet Gynecol 2004;16:447–51.
24. Smith RS, Lauria MR, Comstock CH, et al. Transvaginal ultrasonography for all placentas that appear to be low-lying or over the internal cervical os. Ultrasound Obstet Gynecol 1997;9:22–4.
25. Timor-Tritsch IE, Yunis RA. Confirming the safety of transvaginal sonography in patients suspected of placenta previa. Obstet Gynecol 1993;81:742–4.
26. Nguyen D, Nguyen C, Yacobozzi M, et al. Imaging of the placenta with pathologic correlation. Semin Ultrasound CT MR 2012;33:65–77.
27. Sharma A, Suri V, Gupta I. Tocolytic therapy in conservative management of symptomatic placenta previa. Int J Gynaecol Obstet 2004;84:109–13.
28. Neilson JP. Antenatal corticosteroids for accelerating fetal lung maturation for women at risk of preterm birth. Obstet Gynecol 2007;109:189–90.
29. Roberts D, Dalziel S. Antenatal corticosteroids for accelerating fetal lung maturation for women at risk of preterm birth. Cochrane Database Syst Rev 2006;(3):CD004454.
30. Arias F. Cervical cerclage for the temporary treatment of patients with placenta previa. Obstet Gynecol 1988;71:545–8.
31. Cobo E, Conde-Agudelo A, Delgado J, et al. Cervical cerclage: an alternative for the management of placenta previa? Am J Obstet Gynecol 1998;179:122–5.
32. Neilson JP. Interventions for suspected placenta praevia. Cochrane Database Syst Rev 2003;(2):CD001998.
33. Lang CT, King JC. Maternal mortality in the United States. Best Pract Res Clin Obstet Gynaecol 2008;22:517–31.
34. Conde-Agudelo A, Romero R. Amniotic fluid embolism: an evidence-based review. Am J Obstet Gynecol 2009;201:445.e1–445.e13.
35. Benson MD. Current concepts of immunology and diagnosis in amniotic fluid embolism. Clin Dev Immunol 2012;2012:946576.
36. Clark SL. New concepts of amniotic fluid embolism: a review. Obstet Gynecol Surv 1990;45:360–8.
37. Benson MD. Nonfatal amniotic fluid embolism. Three possible cases and a new clinical definition. Arch Fam Med 1993;2:989–94.
38. Benson MD. A hypothesis regarding complement activation and amniotic fluid embolism. Med Hypotheses 2007;68:1019–25.
39. Fineschi V, Riezzo I, Cantatore S, et al. Complement C3a expression and tryptase degranulation as promising histopathological tests for diagnosing fatal amniotic fluid embolism. Virchows Arch 2009;454:283–90.
40. Kramer MS, Rouleau J, Baskett TF, et al. Amniotic-fluid embolism and medical induction of labour: a retrospective, population-based cohort study. Lancet 2006;368:1444–8.
41. Abenhaim HA, Azoulay L, Kramer MS, et al. Incidence and risk factors of amniotic fluid embolisms: a population-based study on 3 million births in the United States. Am J Obstet Gynecol 2008;199:49.e1–e8.
42. Gist RS, Stafford IP, Leibowitz AB, et al. Amniotic fluid embolism. Anesth Analg 2009;108:1599–602.
43. Clark SL, Hankins GD, Dudley DA, et al. Amniotic fluid embolism: analysis of the national registry. Am J Obstet Gynecol 1995;172:1158–69.

44. Gilbert WM, Danielsen B. Amniotic fluid embolism: decreased mortality in a population-based study. Obstet Gynecol 1999;93:973–7.
45. Burtelow M, Riley E, Druzin M, et al. How we treat: management of life-threatening primary postpartum hemorrhage with a standardized massive transfusion protocol. Transfusion 2007;47:1564–72.
46. Cunningham FG, Leveno KJ, Bloom SL, et al. In: Cunningham FG, Leveno KJ, Bloom SL, editors. Williams obstetrics. 23rd edition. New York: McGraw-Hill Medical; 2010. chapter 36.
47. Henderson S, Mallon W. Labor and delivery and their complications. In: Marx JA, Hockberger RS, Walls RM, et al, editors. Rosen's emergency medicine: concepts and clinical practice. 6th edition. Philadelphia: Mosby/Elsevier; 2006. p. 2798.
48. Di Renzo GC, Roura LC. European Association of Perinatal Medicine-Study Group on Preterm Birth. Guidelines for the management of spontaneous preterm labor. J Perinat Med 2006;34:359–66.
49. Muglia LJ, Katz M. The enigma of spontaneous preterm birth. N Engl J Med 2010; 362:529–35.
50. Martin JA, Hamilton BE, Sutton PD, et al. Births: final data for 2008. Natl Vital Stat Rep 2010;59(1):3–71.
51. Mathews TJ, MacDorman MF. Infant mortality statistics from the 2003 period linked birth/infant death data set. Natl Vital Stat Rep 2006;54:1–29.
52. Von Der Pool BA. Preterm labor: diagnosis and treatment. Am Fam Physician 1998;57:2457–64.
53. Gonik B, Creasy RK. Preterm labor: its diagnosis and management. Am J Obstet Gynecol 1986;154:3–8.
54. Mella MT, Berghella V. Prediction of preterm birth: cervical sonography. Semin Perinatol 2009;33:317–24.
55. Fonseca EB, Celik E, Parra M, et al. Progesterone and the risk of preterm birth among women with a short cervix. N Engl J Med 2007;357:462–9.
56. Gomez R, Galasso M, Romero R, et al. Ultrasonographic examination of the uterine cervix is better than cervical digital examination as a predictor of the likelihood of premature delivery in patients with preterm labor and intact membranes. Am J Obstet Gynecol 1994;171:956–64.
57. Tyson JE, Parikh NA, Langer J, et al. Intensive care for extreme prematurity—moving beyond gestational age. N Engl J Med 2008;358:1672–81.
58. Lockwood CJ, Senyei AE, Dische MR, et al. Fetal fibronectin in cervical and vaginal secretions as a predictor of preterm delivery. N Engl J Med 1991;325: 669–74.
59. Berghella V, Hayes E, Visintine J, et al. Fetal fibronectin testing for reducing the risk of preterm birth. Cochrane Database Syst Rev 2008;(4):CD006843.
60. Di Renzo GC, Roura LC, Facchinetti F, et al. Guidelines for the management of spontaneous preterm labor: identification of spontaneous preterm labor, diagnosis of preterm premature rupture of membranes, and preventive tools for preterm birth. J Matern Fetal Neonatal Med 2011;24:659–67.
61. Practice bulletin No. 127: management of preterm labor. Obstet Gynecol 2012; 119:1308.
62. Haas DM, Imperiale TF, Kirkpatrick PR, et al. Tocolytic therapy: a meta-analysis and decision analysis. Obstet Gynecol 2009;113:585–94.
63. ACOG Committee on Obstetric Practice. ACOG Committee opinion No. 475: antenatal corticosteroid therapy for fetal maturation. Obstet Gynecol 2011;117: 422–4.

64. ACOG Committee on Practice Bulletins-Obstetrics. ACOG practice bulletin No. 80: premature rupture of membranes: clinical management guidelines for obstetrician-gynecologists. Obstet Gynecol 2007;109:1007–19.
65. Moore RM, Mansour JM, Redline RW, et al. The physiology of fetal membrane rupture: insight gained from the determination of physical properties. Placenta 2006;27:1037–51.
66. Mercer BM, Goldenberg RL, Meis PJ, et al. The preterm prediction study: prediction of preterm premature rupture of membranes through clinical findings and ancillary testing. the national institute of child health and human development maternal-fetal medicine units network. Am J Obstet Gynecol 2000;183:738–45.
67. Hadley CB, Main DM, Gabbe SG. Risk factors for preterm premature rupture of the fetal membranes. Am J Perinatol 1990;7:374–9.
68. Hannah ME, Ohlsson A, Farine D, et al. Induction of labor compared with expectant management for prelabor rupture of the membranes at term. TERMPROM study group. N Engl J Med 1996;334:1005–10.
69. Landon MB. Uterine rupture in primigravid women. Obstet Gynecol 2006;108: 709–10.
70. Walsh CA, Baxi LV. Rupture of the primigravid uterus: a review of the literature. Obstet Gynecol Surv 2007;62:327–34 [quiz: 353–4].
71. Porreco RP, Clark SL, Belfort MA, et al. The changing specter of uterine rupture. Am J Obstet Gynecol 2009;200:269.e1–e4.
72. Mirza FG, Gaddipati S. Obstetric emergencies. Semin Perinatol 2009;33:97–103.
73. Dow M, Wax JR, Pinette MG, et al. Third-trimester uterine rupture without previous cesarean: a case series and review of the literature. Am J Perinatol 2009;26: 739–44.
74. Ozdemir I, Yucel N, Yucel O. Rupture of the pregnant uterus: a 9-year review. Arch Gynecol Obstet 2005;272:229–31.
75. Bedi DG, Salmon A, Winsett MZ, et al. Ruptured uterus: sonographic diagnosis. J Clin Ultrasound 1986;14:529–33.
76. Lang CT, Landon MB. Uterine rupture as a source of obstetrical hemorrhage. Clin Obstet Gynecol 2010;53:237–51.

Trauma in Pregnancy

Ali S. Raja, MD, MBA, MPH[a,b,*], Christopher P. Zabbo, DO[c,d,e]

KEYWORDS

- Trauma • Pregnancy • Maternal cardiopulmonary arrest
- Perimortem cesarean section

KEY POINTS

- Pregnant women are at significant risk for injury. Counseling of all pregnant women, regardless of reason for presentation to the emergency department, should include a discussion of seat belt use and screening for domestic violence.
- When treating pregnant trauma victims, the initial focus should be on maternal stability. Any emergent measures necessary to maintain it should be performed, including transfusion (of O-negative blood) and imaging, (even, if needed, emergent computed tomography).
- Follow the basic Advanced Trauma Life Support algorithm: **A**irway, **B**reathing, **C**irculation, **D**isability, and **E**xposure, with uterine displacement (30° to the left) during circulation assessment to increase caval return.
- Once maternal stability has been assured, focus on the fetus (the **F** after **A, B, C, D**, and **E**): placental abruption, uterine rupture, and fetomaternal hemorrhage.
- Continuous fetal monitoring is essential once the mother is stable. If not available, arrange transfer to a facility where it is available. Monitoring should continue for at least 4 hours after the injury if the mother is otherwise asymptomatic but may be continued in patients with regular contractions, continued abdominal pain, vaginal bleeding, or nonreassuring tracings.

INTRODUCTION

The emergency treatment of pregnant patients who sustain trauma requires knowledge of the fundamental aspects of trauma management as well as an understanding of the unique physiologic and anatomic changes of pregnancy that may affect both the

Disclosures and funding sources: Dr Raja: NHLBI, NIBIB, and CMS; Dr Zabbo: None.
Conflict of interest: Dr Raja: None; Dr Zabbo: None.
[a] Department of Emergency Medicine, Brigham and Women's Hospital, 75 Francis Street, Neville House, Boston, MA 02115, USA; [b] Harvard Medical School, 25 Shattuck Street, Boston, MA 02115, USA; [c] Emergency Medicine Residency, Kent Hospital/UNECOM, 455 Toll Gate Road, Warwick, RI 02886, USA; [d] Department of Emergency Medicine, Kent Hospital, 455 Toll Gate Road, Warwick, RI 02886, USA; [e] Department of Emergency Medicine, UNECOM, 11 Hills Beach Road, Biddeford, ME 04005, USA
* Corresponding author. Department of Emergency Medicine, Brigham and Women's Hospital, 75 Francis Street, Neville House, Boston, MA 02115.
E-mail address: asraja@partners.org

Emerg Med Clin N Am 30 (2012) 937–948
http://dx.doi.org/10.1016/j.emc.2012.08.003
emed.theclinics.com

maternal and fetal victims involved. It is important to note that the initial stabilization efforts should focus on ensuring maternal hemodynamic stability because the most common cause of fetal mortality is maternal shock. Once maternal stability is assured, focus can shift to the fetus, unless that initial goal is thought to be unobtainable (see later discussion of perimortem cesarean delivery).

Approximately 7% of pregnant women experience trauma during their pregnancies, with the greatest incidence of trauma occurring within the last trimester. Falls are the most common mechanism of injury (accounting for 51.6% of pregnancy-related injuries in a recent study), and 9.5% of all injuries during pregnancy are intentionally inflicted.[1]

PREVENTION OF INJURY

Although trauma is often unpreventable, the unique aspects of pregnancy and the fact that some emergency department (ED) patients may not seek prenatal care necessitate that emergency physicians treating pregnant patients discuss at least 2 fundamental aspects of injury prevention: domestic violence and seat belt use, regardless of the patients' reasons for visiting the ED.[2]

Domestic violence may either manifest or increase in frequency during pregnancy.[3] Homicide, especially as a result of gunshot wounds caused by firearms, accounts for a significant proportion of prenatal mortality.[4] A recent review found that of penetrating abdominal injuries sustained during pregnancy, 73% occurred as a result of gunshot wounds.[5] Given the significant maternal and fetal mortality associated with domestic violence during pregnancy (3% and 16%, respectively, overall, in this same study), screening is essential. Although obstetric and primary care practices typically use standardized tools that may be too lengthy for the emergency use,[6] even brief domestic violence screening tools have been found to be effective.[7,8]

The other major cause of maternal mortality is blunt trauma, commonly caused by falls and motor vehicle accidents. Although fall prevention is somewhat intuitive, pregnancy-related anatomic changes and their impact on seat belt position should be discussed. The initial focus should be the use of seat belts themselves; a study of pregnant patients involved in motor vehicle accidents found that severe crashes in which the pregnant woman was not wearing a seat belt resulted in adverse outcomes 100% of the time.[9] Once worn, seat belts require correct positioning to prevent force transmission to the uterus and direct uterine trauma; lap belts should pass under (not over or in front of) the gravid uterus, and shoulder belts should pass between the breasts and lateral to the uterus.[10]

THE INITIAL EVALUATION AND MANAGEMENT OF PREGNANT TRAUMA PATIENTS

The initial ED evaluation of all patients with trauma, pregnant or otherwise, should follow the American College of Surgeons Committee on Trauma's Advanced Trauma Life Support guidelines.[11] Maternal stability should be assessed and maintained because this will simultaneously maximize the likelihood of positive maternal and fetal outcomes. In centers with the available resources, obstetric (and neonatal if >24 weeks' estimated gestational age) specialists should be mobilized as early as possible during the evaluation of pregnant trauma patients. It is, however, important to remember that effective team-based care requires coordination by a central team leader, who should be the emergency physician or trauma surgeon primarily responsible for the patient. This leader should in turn ensure appropriate closed-loop communication, prioritization of interventions, and ongoing assessment with the nursing and consultative staff caring for the patient.[12]

Relevant Aspects of Patient History

The focused history obtained during the emergent evaluation of a pregnant patient with trauma should be directed toward clarifying those factors that may alter initial patient management:

- Injury mechanism: Both blunt and penetrating traumas, if intentional, are typically directed toward the abdomen.
- Medications/allergies: Young and otherwise healthy women may develop pregnancy-induced heart failure, gestational diabetes, or venous thromboembolic disease and may be taking medications not otherwise typical in their age group.
- Last menstrual period: If this information is known, it will help determine fetal viability to guide the appropriateness of fetal interventions.
- Fetal movement: Although less important if immediate bedside ultrasonography or fetal monitoring is available, this can serve as a proxy for fetal stability until these objective tests are performed.
- Contractions: Uterine irritability caused by trauma and early labor can necessitate posttraumatic fetal monitoring.
- Abdominal pain/vaginal bleeding/premature rupture of membranes: These situations should prompt a more thorough consideration of trauma-related uterine complications and early labor.

Primary Survey

As with any trauma patient, the primary survey is focused on identifying immediate threats to life and limb. Pregnant trauma patients, however, should have a fetal assessment performed immediately after the maternal primary survey to allow for prompt fetal intervention if appropriate. As mentioned previously, the obstetric service (if available) should be on hand to assist with evaluation and to guide the determination of whether emergent cesarean delivery is indicated.

Airway

The determination of whether a pregnant patient with trauma requires airway intervention necessitates the evaluation of her ability to protect her airway, oxygenate and ventilate, and also a consideration of her anticipated clinical course.[13] It is important to intervene as early as possible, with the understanding that prolonged bag valve mask ventilation of a pregnant patient (who has increased abdominal pressure and decreased lower esophageal tone) significantly increases her risk of aspiration of gastric contents.

It should be anticipated that women in late pregnancy have difficult airways. One study of maternal airways at both 12 and 38 weeks found that that the proportion of Mallampati class 4 airways (with only the hard palate visible and with no view of the soft palate or uvula) increased by 34% between the two periods.[14] The additional fact that these patients have sustained trauma and will likely be in cervical collars simply compounds an already difficult situation.[15] Given this, the use of video laryngoscopy, if available, is paramount because it allows for the maximization of first-pass success in these intubations.[16] Once intubation is accomplished, nasogastric decompression should be performed to minimize the ongoing risk of aspiration.

Breathing

Regardless of whether intubation is needed, supplemental oxygen should be used liberally in pregnant trauma patients. Oxygen consumption increases by almost 20% during pregnancy to meet the increased metabolic demands of the placenta, fetus, and maternal organs.[17] In addition, pregnant women develop a decrease in their functional reserve capacity after 20 weeks, therefore maximizing oxygenation can improve the amount of apneic time tolerable without desaturation if intubation becomes necessary.

Because of the increase in abdominal pressure and elevation of the diaphragm, tube thoracostomy should be performed higher than it would otherwise be performed in nonpregnant patients. Rather than insertion of the chest tube in the fifth or sixth intercostal space, one should use the fourth or fifth intercostal space. If available, bedside ultrasonography can help guide placement of a thoracostomy in pregnant patients with pneumothoraces because the location of the diaphragm on expiration can be directly visualized (**Fig. 1**).

Circulation

A drop in maternal blood pressure can result in decreased placental blood flow and fetal hypoperfusion, making maintenance of maternal blood volume especially important in this patient population. All of these patients should have 2 large bore (14 or 16 gauge) intravenous lines established immediately on their arrival in case emergent transfusion of blood or fluids is needed.

After 20 weeks' gestation, the uterus is large enough to compress the inferior vena cava when pregnant women lie supine. This compression can decrease cardiac output by as much as 30%.[18] It is imperative to displace the uterus of a woman in late pregnancy to the left off of the inferior vena cava, either manually or by tilting the backboard with a wedge or pillow.

In hemodynamically unstable pregnant women, a focused assessment with sonography for trauma (FAST) examination should be performed during the primary survey to assess for possible sources of bleeding. The specificity of FAST in pregnancy has been shown to be similar to that of nonpregnant patients, and positive findings in unstable patients should prompt emergent operative evaluation.[19,20] However, FAST cannot detect retroperitoneal hemorrhage, which is more likely in pregnant women because of the increased blood flow to the uterus.[21]

If a blood transfusion is needed emergently, Rh-negative blood should be used unless the patients' Rh status is known in order to prevent sensitization to Rho(D) factors and erythroblastosis fetalis in subsequent pregnancies.

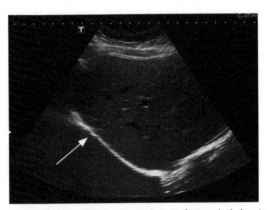

Fig. 1. The appearance of the diaphragm (*arrow*) on a focused abdominal sonography for trauma (FAST) exam. (*From* Roberts HC. Imaging the diaphragm. Thorac Surg Clin 2009; 19(4):431–50; with permission.)

Disability/brief neurologic evaluation
The brief evaluation of disability performed during the primary survey of a pregnant trauma patient does not differ significantly from that of a nonpregnant patient. The examination should be a focused assessment of the patient's level of consciousness using the Glasgow Coma Scale and also an evaluation of their pupillary size, gross motor function, and sensation in each limb. If signs, symptoms, or suspicion of spinal cord injury is present, it is especially important to note any lateralizing signs and the level of intact sensation.

Exposure and environmental control
Given the possibility of domestic violence during pregnancy, it is important to completely evaluate pregnant patients. Be sure to expose and briefly examine all areas of her body, especially the back, because abusers often cause injuries in hidden locations to minimize the risk of discovery. After this initial evaluation, however, ensure that patients are covered and stay dry because hypothermia contributes to coagulopathy, which can be especially detrimental in patients with trauma.[22]

Fetal evaluation
Maternal trauma can result in uterine hypoperfusion and resultant fetal hypotension and hypoxia as well as uterine rupture and placental abruption (discussed later). Fetal monitoring is essential after the primary survey of the mother is complete. If formal continuous fetal monitoring is not available, periodic Doppler measurement or bedside ultrasound calculation of a fetal heart rate is an appropriate temporary substitute. Beware of the potentially tachycardic maternal heart rate in pregnant trauma victims, comparison of the fetal heart rate heard with the Doppler with the maternal pulse on the cardiac monitor can help ensure that it is the fetus's pulse being measured.

In women with viable pregnancies and abdominal trauma, a prolonged period of fetal monitoring is recommended. This monitoring should be for a period of no less than 4 hours and may increase if contractions, vaginal bleeding, abdominal pain, or nonreassuring fetal heart rate variability continues. This monitoring should be performed by the obstetric team in an area conducive to rapid caesarean delivery if fetal distress is noted.[23] The significance of fetal cardiac monitoring after trauma is underscored by a study of 441 pregnant trauma patients, which found that the deaths of 5 infants were caused by delayed recognition of nonreassuring fetal heart rates. Three of these were in only mildly or moderately injured mothers, so these deaths were potentially preventable if the nonreassuring fetal heart rates had been detected early and the patients had gone to emergency cesarean section.[24]

Secondary Survey

The secondary survey of pregnant patients, which involves a more thorough evaluation after hemodynamic stability of both the mother and fetus has been confirmed, is very similar to that in nonpregnant patients. However, specific emphasis should be placed on the abdominal, skin, and vaginal examinations.

Abdomen
In patients who do not know their gestational age, it can be estimated by using the umbilicus as a guide. Fundal height increases by approximately 1 cm above the umbilicus for every week of gestation beyond 20 weeks. This information can be especially useful when determining fetal viability because premature infants born at less than 25 weeks gestational age have extremely high mortality.[25]

In addition, it is important to assess for ecchymoses, especially in blunt trauma. These ecchymoses may be present underneath a gravid uterus (especially late in pregnancy) and may be caused by seat belt injuries, indicating significant abdominal force.

Lastly, tocographic monitoring should be initiated alongside fetal cardiac monitoring because ongoing contractions may necessitate continued evaluation by obstetric specialists.

Skin

Although a cursory examination of the skin for significant evidence of trauma should be performed during the exposure step of the primary survey, the secondary survey allows for a more thorough examination. Specific attention should be paid to the breasts, abdomen, and upper extremities because these can be sites for intentional blunt trauma. Suspicion should be heightened if there are bruises in various states of healing.

Vaginal

The vaginal examination should preferably be performed with an obstetric specialist present. Initial examination should involve a sterile speculum examination to evaluate for vaginal lacerations or bony fragments that may indicate pelvic fractures. If fluid is present, it can be tested for ferning and also for its pH (normal vaginal secretions have a pH of 5.0, whereas amniotic fluid has a pH of 7.0). Bimanual examination should be deferred unless the capability of performing a rapid cesarean section is available because of the possibility of membrane rupture.

USE OF DIAGNOSTIC IMAGING

Given concerns regarding the risks of ionizing radiation (discussed later), the use of X ray and computed tomography (CT) in pregnancy should be minimized, especially if alternative diagnostic modalities (eg, ultrasound or magnetic resonance imaging) may provide similar information. However, in hemodynamically unstable pregnant women with suspected diagnoses for which there are no alternate appropriate studies (eg, those with a suspected retroperitoneal hemorrhage), the benefits of CT imaging far outweigh the fetal risks of radiation, especially given the significant fetal risk of continued uterine hypoperfusion caused by maternal shock. With that caveat in mind, there are 3 main concerns regarding the use of ionizing radiation during pregnancy: loss of viability, radiation-induced malformation, and radiation-induced malignancy.[26] For reference, the typical trauma examinations expose the average patient to the following effective doses: chest X ray (0.002 rad), pelvic X ray (0.06 rad), and abdomen/pelvis CT (1.5 rad).[27,28]

The earliest concern, loss of viability, is greatest when it occurs within 2 weeks of conception, a time period when most pregnant women are unaware that they are pregnant. There is a significant risk of failure to implant with exposure to more than 50 rad of ionizing radiation. However, those embryos that implant should not have significant noncancer health effects.[26]

The risk of radiation-induced malformation is greatest during embryonic organogenesis (2–7 weeks after conception). Although there is no detectable risk with less than 5 rad of exposure, risk of growth retardation increases with more than 5 rad, with growth retardation likely with more than 50 rad of exposure. The risk of malformation decreases later in pregnancy because of the completion of organogenesis.[26]

Although there are little data regarding the risk of in utero ionizing radiation exposure and cancer risk, it is thought to be constant throughout pregnancy. The Centers for Disease Control and Prevention classify the risk as minimal when cumulative exposure during the pregnancy is limited to 0 to 5 rad (<1% risk of malignancy) but state that the risk increases to 1% to 6% when cumulative exposure increases to 5 to 50 rad and more than 6% when cumulative exposure exceeds 50 rad.[26]

In addition to the decision of when to use imaging, it is important to remember that certain pregnancy-related anatomic changes may seem to be abnormalities on plain imaging routinely obtained during trauma. Chest radiographs may have slight cardiomegaly, a slightly widened mediastinum, and mild pulmonary vascular cephalization, whereas pelvis radiographs may have widening of the sacroiliac joints and the symphysis pubis, both of which occur normally in pregnancy.

TRAUMATIC COMPLICATIONS OF PREGNANCY
Placental Abruption

While placental abruption can occur spontaneously, it is most often described in the setting of trauma, especially abdominal trauma. One case series noted that the incidence of abruption increased with the severity of injury, from 8.5% in noninjured pregnant women involved in car accidents to 13% in women with severe injuries.[29] Although the diagnosis is classically made based on the presence of abdominal pain, uterine tenderness, or vaginal bleeding, it can also be present in asymptomatic mothers. Ultrasound is also not sensitive enough to rule out abruption, necessitating the use of routine posttraumatic fetal cardiac and tocographic monitoring.[30]

Uterine Rupture

Both blunt and penetrating trauma can cause uterine rupture, and the diagnosis should always be considered in pregnant trauma patients with a significant mechanism of injury. Although pregnant patients are typically counseled to avoid placing their seat belts directly over their uterus, inappropriate seat belt placement can result in significant force directed directly on the uterus. In addition, intentional penetrating trauma is often directed at the uterus in pregnant women, putting them at greater risk for uterine rupture. In contrast to nonpregnant patients for whom operative intervention is typically appropriate after penetrating trauma, pregnant women with lower abdominal penetrating trauma may be treated more conservatively given the superior displacement of other abdominal organs by the uterus. Pregnant women with upper abdominal trauma, on the other hand, are typically taken for operative evaluation similar to their nonpregnant counterparts.[18,31]

Fetomaternal Hemorrhage

Fetomaternal hemorrhage (FMH) causes alloimmunization in Rh-negative mothers gestating Rh-positive fetuses. Fetal blood that leaks into the maternal circulation following trauma poses a significant concern to the fetus, which results in hemolytic disease of the newborn, fetal anemia, fetal distress, and fetal death.[32] FMH should be considered a possible sequelae of trauma in pregnant patients as early as the fourth week of gestation when the fetal circulation develops. As little as 0.1 mL of fetal blood is needed to sensitize the mother.

The Kleihauer-Betke test is an inexpensive, readily available test to measure the percent of fetal red blood cells in a maternal blood sample. The test is sensitive enough to detect 5 mL of FMH. Because less than 5 mL is required to sensitize the mother, all Rh-negative pregnant patients having sustained abdominal trauma should receive Rh immune globulin (RhIG). A 50-µg dose of RhIG is used during the first trimester. After 12 weeks' gestation, a RhIG dose of 300 µg is recommended. The test is useful when it detects greater than 30 mL of FMH, which requires increased doses of RhIG. A positive Kleihauer-Betke test can be combined with other parameters, such as third trimester trauma, abdominal trauma, and an Injury Severity Score greater than 2, to create a composite morbidity model to identify those at risk for adverse perinatal outcomes.[33]

The Kleihauer-Betke test cannot be used to detect FMH in Rh-positive mothers or in Rh-negative mothers carrying an Rh-negative fetus. Although alloimmunization and hemolytic disease of the newborn are not a concern, significant FMH may lead to fetal exsanguination. Uterine tenderness, contractions, vaginal bleeding, and fetal distress may indicate FMH. Current research is looking at anti–fetal hemoglobin flow cytometry as an alternative to detecting FMH.[34]

PERIMORTEM CESAREAN SECTION

In the cardiopulmonary arrest of pregnant trauma patients, the emergency medicine physician must consider the survivability of both the mother and the fetus. The best chance of fetal survival is maternal survival, and the best chance of maternal survival may be fetal delivery. The perimortem cesarean section relieves the aortocaval compression, which will improve the effectiveness of cardiopulmonary resuscitation (CPR). This relief increases cardiac output by approximately 60% to 80%.[35] The 2010 American Heart Association (AHA) guidelines recommend cesarean delivery if maternal resuscitative efforts are not successful by 4 minutes. There have been a few case reports and no clinical trials regarding perimortem cesarean section; however, between 1900 and 1985, the case reports showed that normal neurologic outcome in the fetus was more likely with delivery within 5 minutes of the mothers' arrest.[36] From these case reports, the 5-minute rule was established. Between 1985 and 2004, the case reports show that 12 out of 20 mothers had improved hemody-namics or return of spontaneous circulation with perimortem cesarean section.[37] These same case reports continue to establish that the likelihood of normal neurologic outcome in the fetus relies on delivery within 5 minutes of maternal arrest, with 9 out of 12 infants delivered within that time showing normal neurologic function.[38] It should be noted that the case reports and subsequent AHA guidelines focus on medical causes of maternal cardiac arrest. Traumatic hypovolemic cardiac arrest in a mother portends a worse outcome for the fetus because the fetus has already suffered prolonged hypoxia.

Another factor to consider before performing the perimortem cesarean section is gestational age. It is thought that aortocaval compression begins to occur at 20 weeks' gestation. Most institutions will provide full support to a fetus between 22 and 24 weeks' gestation. The 2010 AHA guidelines state that, with an obvious gravid uterus and no return of spontaneous circulation by 4 minutes, a perimortem cesarean section should be performed. The perimortem cesarean section is a reasonable option when the fetus is estimated to be 22 to 24 weeks' gestation with the best information available or the uterus is at or above the umbilicus.

During the procedure, CPR should be continued and broad-spectrum antibiotics should be given to decrease any risk of postpartum infection. The most experienced physician, preferably an obstetrician, should perform the cesarean section; but because of the time constraints in which the procedure must be performed, the responsibility will likely be that of the emergency medicine physician or trauma surgeon. A neonatologist or pediatrician should be requested to the resuscitation room immediately, but this should not delay the procedure. The suggested incision is a vertical incision from the epigastrium to the symphysis pubis and carried through all layers to the peritoneal cavity (**Fig. 2**), which provides a fast entry and adequate visualization of the uterus. The uterus is exposed and initially incised at the bladder

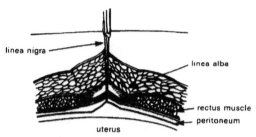

Fig. 2. The abdominal incision for a perimortem cesarean section. (*From* Strong TH, Lowe RA. Perimortem cesarean section. Am J Emer Med 1989;7(5):489–94; with permission.)

reflection, with a retractor pulling the bladder caudally (**Fig. 3**). The incision should then be extended to the uterine fundus, with the operator's hand used to palpate for fetal parts and prevent them from being damaged by the scissors being used to extend the incision (**Fig. 4**). The infant should be extracted with prompt clamping and cutting of the umbilical cord.

The physician is now faced with the resuscitation of 2 separate patients. With maternal CPR continuing, if hemodynamic stability is restored with the relief of venal compression, delivery of the placenta and closure of the uterus should be performed to limit further hemorrhage. The infant should be managed according to the 2010 AHA/ American Academy of Pediatrics/International Liaison Committee on Resuscitation's guidelines for neonatal resuscitative care. Additional resources (pediatric and obstetric/surgical) should be called and divided to continue both resuscitations; but if resources are limited or unavailable, the physician may need to focus on the patient deemed to have the greatest chance of survival.

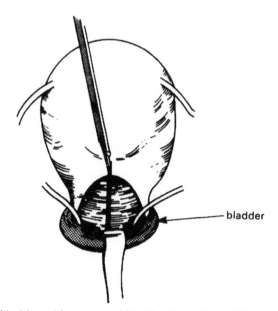

Fig. 3. The initial incision with a retracted bladder. (*From* Strong TH, Lowe RA. Perimortem cesarean section. Am J Emer Med 1989;7(5):489–94; with permission.)

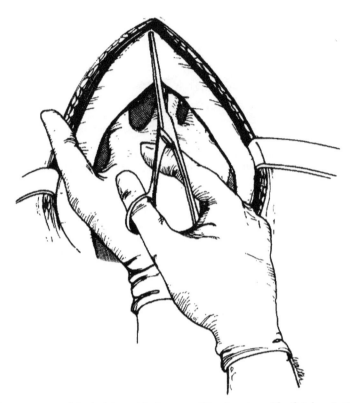

Fig. 4. The extension of the incision with the noncutting hand used for fetal protection. (*From* Strong TH, Lowe RA. Perimortem cesarean section. Am J Emer Med 1989;7(5):489–94; with permission.)

SUMMARY

Trauma, both intentional and unintentional, is a significant cause of maternal morbidity and mortality. All pregnant women evaluated in the ED, regardless of their reason for the visit, should receive trauma prevention focused counseling. Although the initial treatment of pregnant trauma victims should follow the standard protocols of Advanced Trauma Life Support, knowledge about maternal anatomic differences (especially regarding uterine compression of the inferior vena cava) is essential. Fetal stability should be monitored via continuous fetal cardiac monitoring, and an emergent cesarean section may be indicated if this fetal monitoring is thought to be nonreassuring in a viable fetus.

REFERENCES

1. Tinker SC, Reefhuis J, Dellinger AM, et al. Epidemiology of maternal injuries during pregnancy in a population-based study, 1997-2005. J Womens Health (Larchmt) 2010;19(12):2211–8.
2. Kothari CL, Wendt A, Liggins O, et al. Assessing maternal risk for fetal-infant mortality: a population-based study to prioritize risk reduction in a healthy start community. Matern Child Health J 2011;15(1):68–76.

3. Stewart DE. Incidence of postpartum abuse in women with a history of abuse during pregnancy. CMAJ 1994;151(11):1601–4.
4. Chang J, Berg CJ, Saltzman LE, et al. Homicide: a leading cause of injury deaths among pregnant and postpartum women in the United States, 1991-1999. Am J Public Health 2005;95(3):471–7.
5. Petrone P, Talving P, Browder T, et al. Abdominal injuries in pregnancy: a 155-month study at two level 1 trauma centers. Injury 2011;42(1):47–9.
6. Hillard PJ. Physical abuse in pregnancy. Obstet Gynecol 1985;66(2):185–90.
7. McFarlane J, Parker B, Soeken K, et al. Assessing for abuse during pregnancy. Severity and frequency of injuries and associated entry into prenatal care. JAMA 1992;267(23):3176–8.
8. Krimm J, Heinzer MM. Domestic violence screening in the emergency department of an urban hospital. J Natl Med Assoc 2002;94(6):484.
9. Pearlman MD, Phillips ME. Safety belt use during pregnancy. Obstet Gynecol 1996;88(6):1026–9.
10. Pearlman MD, Viano D. Automobile crash simulation with the first pregnant crash test dummy. Am J Obstet Gynecol 1996;175(4 Pt 1):977–81.
11. American College of Surgeons Committee on Trauma. Advanced trauma life support for doctors, student course manual. 8th edition. Chicago: American College of Surgeons; 2008.
12. Szyld D, Peyre S, Cooper Z, et al. MedEdPORTAL. Trauma team training: multidisciplinary training for trauma management. Available at: https://www.mededportal. org/publication/8267. Accessed June 29, 2012.
13. Walls R, Murphy M. Manual of emergency airway management. 3rd edition. Philadelphia: Lippincott Williams & Wilkins; 2008.
14. Pilkington S, Carli F, Dakin MJ, et al. Increase in Mallampati score during pregnancy. Br J Anaesth 1995;74(6):638–42.
15. Sakles JC, Josephy CP, Chiu SF. Success rates of Glidescope® video laryngoscopy versus direct laryngoscopy in blunt trauma patients with cervical immobilization. J Emerg Med 2009;37(2):220.
16. Maruyama K, Yamada T, Kawakami R, et al. Randomized cross-over comparison of cervical-spine motion with the Airway Scope or Macintosh laryngoscope with in-line stabilization: a video-fluoroscopic study. Br J Anaesth 2008;101(4):563–7.
17. Prowse CM, Gaensler EA. Respirator and acid-base changes during pregnancy. Anesthesiology 1965;26:381–92.
18. Muench MV, Canterino JC. Trauma in pregnancy. Obstet Gynecol Clin North Am 2007;34(3):555–83, xiii.
19. Goodwin H, Holmes JF, Wisner DH. Abdominal ultrasound examination in pregnant blunt trauma patients. J Trauma 2001;50(4):689–93 [discussion: 694].
20. Richards JR, Ormsby EL, Romo MV, et al. Blunt abdominal injury in the pregnant patient: detection with US. Radiology 2004;233(2):463–70.
21. Stone IK. Trauma in the obstetric patient. Obstet Gynecol Clin North Am 1999; 26(3):459–67, viii.
22. Hess JR, Brohi K, Dutton RP, et al. The coagulopathy of trauma: a review of mechanisms. J Trauma 2008;65(4):748–54.
23. Esposito TJ. Trauma during pregnancy. Emerg Med Clin North Am 1994;12(1): 167–99.
24. Morris JA Jr, Rosenbower TJ, Jurkovich GJ, et al. Infant survival after cesarean section for trauma. Ann Surg 1996;223(5):481–8 [discussion: 488–91].
25. El-Metwally D, Vohr B, Tucker R. Survival and neonatal morbidity at the limits of viability in the mid 1990s: 22 to 25 weeks. J Pediatrics 2000;137(5):616–22.

26. CDC radiation emergencies and prenatal radiation exposure: a fact sheet for physicians. Available at: http://www.bt.cdc.gov/radiation/prenatalphysician.asp. Accessed June 29, 2012.
27. Mettler FA Jr, Huda W, Yoshizumi TT, et al. Effective doses in radiology and diagnostic nuclear medicine: a catalog. Radiology 2008;248(1):254–63.
28. Smith-Bindman R, Lipson J, Marcus R, et al. Radiation dose associated with common computed tomography examinations and the associated lifetime attributable risk of cancer. Arch Intern Med 2009;169(22):2078–86.
29. Schiff MA, Holt VL. Pregnancy outcomes following hospitalization for motor vehicle crashes in Washington State from 1989 to 2001. Am J Epidemiol 2005; 161(6):503–10.
30. Kuhlmann RS, Warsof S. Ultrasound of the placenta. Clin Obstet Gynecol 1996; 39(3):519–34.
31. Awwad JT, Azar GB, Seoud MA, et al. High-velocity penetrating wounds of the gravid uterus: review of 16 years of civil war. Obstet Gynecol 1994;83(2):259–64.
32. Pearlman MD, Tintinalli JE, Lorenz RP. Blunt trauma during pregnancy. N Engl J Med 1990;323(23):1609–13.
33. Trivedi N, Ylagan M, Moore TR, et al. Predicting adverse outcomes following trauma in pregnancy. J Reprod Med 2012;57(1–2):3–8.
34. Kim YA, Makar RS. Detection of fetomaternal hemorrhage. Am J Hematology 2012;87(4):417–23.
35. Hill CC, Pickinpaugh J. Trauma and surgical emergencies in the obstetric patient. Surg Clin North Am 2008;88(2):421–40, viii.
36. Katz VL, Dotters DJ, Droegemueller W. Perimortem cesarean delivery. Obstet Gynecol 1986;68(4):571–6.
37. DePace NL, Betesh JS, Kotler MN. "Postmortem" cesarean section with recovery of both mother and offspring. JAMA 1982;248(8):971–3.
38. Katz V, Balderston K, DeFreest M. Perimortem cesarean delivery: were our assumptions correct? Am J Obstet Gynecol 2005;192(6):1916–20 [discussion: 1920–21].

Cardiovascular Disasters in Pregnancy

Sarah K. Sommerkamp, MD, RDMS*, Alisa Gibson, MD, DMD

KEYWORDS

- Pregnancy • Pulmonary embolus • Aortic dissection • Cardiomyopathy
- Acute myocardial infarction • Arrhythmia • Cardiac arrest
- Perimortem cesarean section

KEY POINTS

- During pregnancy, the D-dimer level is likely to be elevated; however, a negative D-dimer is still reliably negative in a patient with low pretest probability.
- Life-threatening pulmonary embolism can be treated with tissue plasminogen activator, despite the relative contraindication of pregnancy.
- Aortic dissection is more common in pregnancy and in the immediate postpartum period than their nonpregnant counterparts.
- Cardiac disease in pregnancy is becoming more common, because of the increasing incidence of advanced maternal age, obesity, hypertension, and diabetes mellitus and improved treatments for congenital heart disease.
- Percutaneous coronary intervention is first-line therapy for pregnant patients with acute myocardial infarction.
- Displacement of the uterus is imperative to a successful resuscitation.
- Drug and electricity doses are unchanged in resuscitation of the pregnant patient.
- Perimortem cesarean section must be completed within 5 minutes of loss of circulation.

INTRODUCTION

The normal changes that occur during pregnancy are demanding on the cardiovascular system. Total cardiac output increases about 50% from a combination of increased blood volume and pulse along with a decrease in peripheral resistance. These changes can place significant stress on a normal heart. Physiologic changes are even more dangerous to individuals with underlying cardiac disorders. Cardiac arrest can occur in previously asymptomatic women who are experiencing this type of cardiac stress. In its 2010 guidelines,[1] the American Heart Association summarized

Funding sources: None.
Conflict of interest: None.
Department of Emergency Medicine, University of Maryland School of Medicine, 6th Floor, Suite 200, 110 South Paca Street, Baltimore, MD 21201, USA
* Corresponding author.
E-mail address: ssommerkamp@gmail.com

Emerg Med Clin N Am 30 (2012) 949–959
http://dx.doi.org/10.1016/j.emc.2012.08.007
0733-8627/12/$ – see front matter © 2012 Elsevier Inc. All rights reserved.
emed.theclinics.com

the scope of cardiac arrest in pregnancy, citing figures from the Confidential Enquiries into Maternal and Child Health data set[2]: "The overall maternal mortality rate was calculated at 13.95 deaths per 100 000 maternities. There were 8 cardiac arrests with a frequency calculated at 0.05 per 1000 maternities, or 1:20,000." The report notes that the frequency of cardiac arrest during pregnancy is rising. Despite being younger and healthier than many patients with cardiac arrest, pregnant women have more dismal outcomes than their nonpregnant counterparts. One case series described a survival rate of only 6.9%.[3] Many cardiopulmonary pathologies can lead to the endpoint of cardiac arrest during pregnancy. The most significant of these are discussed in this article.

VENOUS THROMBOEMBOLISM

Venous thromboembolism (VTE) is significantly more common in pregnancy, than in nonpregnant women. The number of deaths from thrombosis and thromboembolism is estimated at 1.94 per 100,000 pregnancies.[1] Pregnancy in general is a hypercoagulable state, and certain conditions in pregnant women (eg, lupus anticoagulant and antiphospholipid syndrome) can increase the risk of VTE even further. Diagnosis of deep vein thrombosis (DVT) and pulmonary embolism (PE) is more challenging in pregnancy, because standard tests may be unreliable or dangerous.

D-dimer, a blood test used to aid in the diagnosis of DVT and PE, represents a breakdown product of cross-linked fibrin. It is highly sensitive but lacks specificity in healthy, nonpregnant individuals. During pregnancy, it becomes even less specific. A negative D-dimer is still reliably negative in a patient with low pretest probability, but is a result that is less likely to be obtained. This is because the D-dimer level is usually elevated in normal pregnancies. It typically rises throughout pregnancy, peaking around the time of delivery. Although reported rates of negative D-dimer throughout the stages of pregnancy vary widely, it is clear that the usefulness of the D-dimer to rule out VTE decreases as pregnancy progresses.[4–6] An alternative strategy is to use "trimester-adjusted" D-dimer value to rule out VTE. Kline and associates[4] proposed threshold values of 750 ng/dL in the first trimester, 1000 ng/dL in the second, and 1250 ng/dL in the third. The trimester-adjusted D-dimer measurement is a promising theory that has not yet been tested.

Imaging in pregnancy is obviously problematic because of the goal of avoiding exposure of the mother and fetus to radiation. Diagnosing DVT is still relatively straightforward because ultrasound confers no radiation. This test is an excellent starting point even if PE is the primary concern. If DVT is present, the treatment decision has been made, and there is no need for computed tomography (CT) or ventilation/perfusion (V/Q) scan. After the patient is hospitalized, an echocardiogram can be obtained to assess for complications of PE. However, a negative ultrasound cannot definitively rule out DVT because pelvic DVT is more common in pregnancy than in the nonpregnant state and is likely to be missed on ultrasound. In addition, a negative ultrasound in no way rules out PE.

The use of CT versus V/Q for diagnosis of PE is a matter of perennial debate. The data are quite clear, although the optimal decision is less so. Helical CT delivers radiation to the woman, which is of added concern given the sensitivity of the breast tissue during pregnancy. However, CT exposes the fetus to significantly less radiation. One study found that in the third trimester (when the radiation dose to the fetus is highest), helical CT delivers 0.13 mGy, V/Q scanning 0.37 mGy, and pulmonary arteriography 0.50 mGy.[7] Perfusion scanning has the advantage of delivering 30 to 40 times less radiation to the breast tissue. This is particularly relevant in young, pregnant women, whose breasts have a high cell turnover rate and are highly susceptible to the effects of ionizing radiation.[8] One study of 205 pregnant patients found equivalent negative predictive values (99%–100%) for CT and V/Q. Of the patients who underwent CT, 13% had other clinically significant abnormalities.[9] The bottom line is this: V/Q scan exposes the mother to less radiation but exposes the fetus to more. CT may reveal alternate pathology. The dose of radiation for both is within "acceptable" limits. However, given that any amount of radiation increases the lifetime risk of cancer, the decision must be made on a case-by-case basis. For example, in a patient at higher-than-average risk for breast cancer, a V/Q scan may be the better choice. The patient must be involved in the discussion and given information in a clear, factual manner.

Magnetic resonance imaging (MRI) is emerging as another tool for the diagnosis of PE.[10] The obvious advantage is its lack of ionizing radiation. Disadvantages include the length of time that an ill, unstable patient needs to be away from the emergency department (ED); the need for the patient to lie supine (potentially problematic in a pregnant patient, because of compression of the inferior vena cava); and the uncertainty of the effects of MRI on the fetus. No harmful effects to the fetus have been reported in magnetic fields up to 1.5 T.[11,12] At this point, clinical data regarding the sensitivity and specificity of MRI for PE remain limited, so MRI should not be used to definitively exclude this condition.

After PE has been diagnosed, additional testing including electrocardiography, measurement of troponin, and echocardiography is indicated, as with nonpregnant patients. If these tests show massive PE, administration of tissue plasminogen activator can be considered on a case-by-case basis.

After the definitive diagnosis of DVT or submassive PE has been made, there are two treatment options. Heparin has been used traditionally and is a category C drug in pregnancy. However, it has significant drawbacks, including the need for a drip, frequent blood draws, and therefore hospitalization. Its major use is when delivery is imminent and greater control is desired. Lovenox, a low-molecular-weight heparin and a category B drug, has largely replaced heparin for long-term treatment of thrombotic disease. Coumadin is one of the few category X drugs, capable of producing a teratogenic syndrome. This drug must not be prescribed to pregnant women. Although pregnancy is a relative contraindication for the administration of tissue plasminogen activator, in the setting of cardiac arrest, it might be an appropriate intervention. The successful use of fibrinolytics in pregnant women has been reported for massive, life-threatening PE[13–15] and ischemic stroke.[16] Despite the lack of specific data in pregnancy, pregnant women in cardiac arrest with suspected PE should be treated in accordance with Advanced Cardiovascular Life Support (ACLS) guidelines. These state that in patients in cardiac arrest with known or presumed PE, thrombolytics improve survival to discharge and neurologic outcomes, despite the increased potential for bleeding.[17–19]

AORTIC DISSECTION

Aortic dissection is the second most common cause of maternal death.[1] It is more common than venous thromboembolic disease and occurs more commonly during pregnancy or the immediate postpartum period. Half of the dissections in women younger than 40 occur during pregnancy.[20] Arterial dissections are thought to be related to hormonal and hemodynamic effects on the intima and media of the arterial wall.[21,22]

The diagnosis is challenging, for the same reasons discussed in the VTE section. The D-dimer level is often used as a screening tool, but its reliability has not been validated in nonpregnant patients and its use becomes more complex given the higher baseline levels during pregnancy, as previously discussed. Imaging is required for definitive diagnosis of aortic dissection. As in nonpregnant patients, CT, MRI, and transesophageal electrocardiography (TEE) can be used. Transabdominal ultrasound sometimes shows, but does not reliably exclude, dissection. The gravid abdomen makes this examination even more challenging. TEE is ideal if it is available, because it avoids radiation and can be done in the ED or operating room and has no associated radiation. CT with intravenous contrast is an effective diagnostic tool but delivers a large dose of radiation and the intravenous contrast material. MRI is problematic for any patient with a dissection, because of the length of the study and the location of the imaging suite outside the ED, but it does have the advantage of no radiation. In most hospitals, where TEE is frequently not immediately available, CT becomes the test of choice. Treatment focuses on reducing blood pressure and pulse to decrease shear stress on the aorta. β-Blockers are generally considered safe in pregnancy (**Table 1**). Treatment is the same as for nonpregnant patients, including antihypertensives and vascular or cardiothoracic surgery. An obstetrician should be consulted to monitor fetal well-being.

CARDIAC DISEASE

According to the Confidential Enquiries into Maternal and Child Health report, cardiac disease accounts for 2.27 deaths per 100,000 pregnancies and its incidence has been increasing since 1991.[2] Acquired heart disease complicates 1% to 4% of pregnancies and causes a significant amount of morbidity and mortality. In the developing world (and among immigrants living in Western countries), mitral stenosis from rheumatic fever is the predominant cause. In the United States, congenital heart disease is much more common, likely because of the quality of medical care, which enables these patients to survive past childhood. In addition, the prevalence of obesity, hypertension, diabetes, and hypercholesterolemia in the United States increases the frequency of coronary artery disease. As the number of pregnancies in women at an advanced maternal age continues to rise, this issue is becoming ever more relevant.

Table 1 Select cardiac drugs in pregnancy		
Action	**Medication**	**Considerations**
Afterload reduction	Hydralazine	Often chosen first in pregnancy
	Nitrates	Commonly used and considered safe, but pose a theoretic risk of cyanide toxicity (nitroprusside)
	ACE inhibitors	CANNOT be used in pregnancy, but first choice in postpartum patients
Preload	Loop diuretics	Most likely necessary
	Nitrates	Commonly used and considered safe, but pose a theoretic risk of cyanide toxicity (nitroprusside)
β-Blockers	Metoprolol	Considered safe; some evidence of IUGR
Vasopressors	Dobutamine	Best studied in pregnancy
Antiarrhythmics	Adenosine	No clear evidence, presumed safe
	Amiodarone	Reports of fetal thyroid and neurologic abnormalities
	Procainamide	No clear evidence, considered safer than amiodarone
	Verapamil	Does not pose large risk

Abbreviations: ACE, angiotensin-converting enzyme; IUGR, intrauterine growth retardation.
Data from Refs.[50–52]

When evaluating patients with cardiac disease in the ED, it is helpful to understand the conditions that are most likely to lead to poor maternal and fetal outcomes. A prospective study of 562 women with 617 pregnancies validated four predictors of cardiac events (**Table 2**).[23] The presence or absence of these risk factors should never be given precedence over the clinical picture, but they should be viewed as a "red flag" for a patient with the potential to rapidly deteriorate. Specific problems that merit discussion include valvular problems, cardiomyopathy, and acute myocardial infarction (AMI).

Valvular diseases that complicate pregnancy have structural and infectious origins. Not surprisingly, the degree of risk to mother and fetus increases with the severity of valvular dysfunction. Most adverse events occur in patients with moderate to severe mitral or aortic stenosis.[24] Infective endocarditis is a rare but potentially lethal disease in the setting of pregnancy. The risk factors are similar to those in nonpregnant patients.[25]

Cardiomyopathy in young women may be caused by a viral infection (including HIV); toxicologic sources (alcohol, cocaine, doxorubicin); pregnancy itself (peripartum cardiomyopathy), or, less commonly, ischemia induced by coronary artery disease. Women with ejection fractions less than 40% to 45% are at the highest risk.[26,27] Although some patients present with a known diagnosis of cardiomyopathy, the astute emergency physician must maintain a high level of suspicion for this diagnosis in the pregnant patient with dyspnea, fatigue, and pedal edema. The challenge is that these signs and symptoms are frequently present in normal, healthy pregnancies. Further compounding the diagnostic challenge, multiple other conditions can lead to similar symptoms, including pulmonary causes (asthma, PE); infection (pneumonia); cardiac (AMI); anemia; and preeclampsia. The differential diagnosis can be narrowed in large part by the history and physical examination. Ancillary tests, including electrocardiography, imaging, and laboratory studies, also are frequently required.

Brain natriuretic peptide (BNP) may be helpful in ruling in or out a diagnosis of decompensated heart failure. BNP is secreted by the heart when it is overworked, as occurs in cardiac failure. A value less than 100 pg/mL is considered normal, effectively excluding decompensated heart failure. Values between 100 pg/mL and 300 pg/mL indicate potential cardiac disease, whereas values greater than 300 pg/mL indicate the presence of congestive heart failure.[28] Although the BNP level doubles during a normal pregnancy, in part because of increased blood volume, the value should still be less than 100 pg/mL.[29] BNP may have predictive value beyond aiding with the differentiation of the causes of dyspnea. Tanous and colleagues[30] used the BNP value to predict adverse events from a cardiac cause in pregnant women. They determined

Table 2	
Predictors of cardiac events in patients with acquired heart disease	
Risk Factor	**Point Value**
New York Heart Association Class II–IV heart failure or cyanosis	1
Previous cardiac event (CVA, TIA, ACS) or arrhythmia	1
Left heart obstruction (MV area <2 cm², AV area <1.5 cm², peak LV outflow gradient >30 mm Hg)	1
Ejection fraction <40%	1

Abbreviations: ACS, acute coronary syndrome; AV, aortic valve; CVA, cerebrovascular accident; LV, left ventricular; MV, mitral valve; TIA, transient ischemic attack.
   Risk of cardiac event: 0 points, 4%; 1 point, 26%; >1 point, 62%.
   Data from Siu SC, Sermer M, Colman JM, et al. Prospective multicenter study of pregnancy outcomes in women with heart disease. Circulation 2001;104:515–21.

that a BNP value greater than 100 pg/mL is a sensitive (but not specific) predictor of cardiac events. They also noted patients at greatest risk were those with left ventricular dysfunction.[30]

Management of the pregnant patient with cardiomyopathy depends on the severity of the disease. In general, the approach is the same as for nonpregnant patients with heart failure. Data supporting any particular treatment regimen are limited. Severe diseases may require intervention to control the airway. Noninvasive ventilation strategies should be considered early and may help to avoid intubation. Medication strategies are aimed at reducing afterload and increasing pump function. Although the safety of various medications during pregnancy must be considered (see **Table 1**), the drugs that should be used are essentially unchanged. The major exception is that angiotensin-converting enzyme (ACE) inhibitors are absolutely contraindicated in pregnancy. Patients with decompensated heart failure require admission to the hospital, and obstetrics and cardiology should be consulted early.

Among women of reproductive age, AMI occurs three to four times more often in those who are pregnant versus those who are not pregnant.[31] Management is essentially unchanged in pregnancy. One major exception is thrombolysis, which is relatively contraindicated in pregnancy. Percutaneous coronary intervention (PCI) is first-line therapy for patients with ST-elevation AMI.[32] If PCI is not available at the treating facility, strong consideration should be given to transfer after discussion with a cardiologist, an obstetrician, and the patient. Aspirin,[33,34] β-blockers,[35,36] and nitrates[37] can all be used. Heparin does not cross the placenta, but careful consideration should be given to its use in patients with potential for severe bleeding (placenta previa or abruption, threatened miscarriage).[38] Clopidogrel is generally considered safe, but it causes a significant bleeding risk during delivery.[38] Statins, ACE inhibitors, and angiotensin II receptor blockers are absolutely contraindicated and should all be postponed until after delivery.[39]

Cardiac disease in pregnancy encompasses a huge spectrum of pathologic conditions. However, their management is very similar to that used in nonpregnant patients. Key differences include avoidance of ACE inhibitors in patients with decompensated heart failure and PCI instead of thrombolysis if it is available. Involve consultants early and intervene aggressively, remembering that the health of the fetus depends on a healthy mother.

CARDIAC DYSRHYTHMIAS

Of all the dangerous cardiac conditions discussed, dysrhythmias are the most commonly encountered during pregnancy.[23,40] They occur in women with structurally normal hearts and in women with cardiac abnormalities. Palpitations are a frequent presenting complaint, and the work-up for many of those patients is benign. However, life-threatening dysrhythmias must be excluded. The precise cause of the high frequency is unclear, but the increased stress put on the heart by hormonal and hemodynamic shifts seems to be contributing factors. In addition, thyroid disease is more common during pregnancy than in the nonpregnant state. The source of cardiac dysrhythmia usually can be diagnosed through the history and electrocardiography alone. In some patients, prolonged monitoring and echocardiography are required.

Diagnosis of dysrhythmia generally warrants consultation with a cardiologist and an obstetrician. In general, dysrhythmias in a pregnant woman are managed the same way as in a nonpregnant patient. The exception is in the choice of medication; many antiarrhythmic drugs are teratogenic.

Supraventricular tachycardia is common in pregnancy. Adenosine can be used safely in usual doses. Atrial fibrillation can be managed with rhythm control, rate control, or cardioversion.[41]

Cardioversion is considered safe in all stages of pregnancy.[42–44] Dysrhythmia in the fetus is rare but reported, so a viable fetus should be monitored.[45] Sedation should be used during cardioversion, but during the third trimester it increases the risk of aspiration, airway edema, and decreased functional reserve capacity, causing rapid hypoxia. Cardioversion in the operating room should be considered. If the duration of atrial fibrillation is uncertain or more than 48 hours, low-molecular-weight heparin is preferred for anticoagulation. If antiarrhythmic drugs are required, there are very few data to recommend one drug over another (see **Table 1**). Virtually all of these drugs cross the placenta. Indications for temporary or permanent pacing in patients with symptomatic bradycardias are the same as in nonpregnant patients, and transcutaneous and transvenous pacing can be used.[46]

CARDIAC ARREST

Cardiac arrest during pregnancy has many possible causes, including all of the disease states discussed previously. Initial management includes obtaining intravenous access above the diaphragm, administering 100% oxygen, and relieving compression of the inferior vena cava. Aortocaval compression can be relieved by several methods. The gravid uterus can be displaced manually by either a one-handed push from the patient's right side or a two-handed pull from the left. A left lateral tilt can be created by placing a wedge under a backboard, with a goal angle of 30 degrees (such that the patient does not slide off the board). Effective cardiac compressions can be delivered with this patient positioning. These techniques for uterine displacement improve maternal hemodynamics.[1]

The importance of effective cardiac compression is highlighted in the recent guidelines that changed the long-standing resuscitation algorithm from the ABCs to the C, A, B.[47] When cardiac compressions need to be administered to a pregnant patient, the gravid uterus can interfere with the procedure and upwardly displace the internal organs. Therefore, the location for delivery of effective compressions needs to change: compressions should be delivered slightly higher on the sternum.[1]

The pregnant patient's airway undergoes significant physiologic changes and exhibits increased mucosal edema, secretions, and friability, which are important to recognize because they can lead to a potentially difficult airway. Progesterone decreases sphincter tone, and upward displacement of the abdominal organs increases the risk of aspiration. Breathing is affected by the upward shift of the diaphragm, leading to a decrease in functional residual capacity, intrapulmonary shunting, increased metabolic demand, and thus faster desaturation.

Defibrillation should not be delayed in the coding pregnant patient. Doses for defibrillation are unchanged from the recommended ACLS doses for the non-pregnant patients.[1] Although case reports have described potential harm to the fetus and induction of fatal fetal arrhythmias from high doses of electricity, in a dead or dying patient, these theoretic risks in no way override the benefit of standard defibrillation practices. If fetal monitoring is in place when cardiac arrest occurs, it is reasonable to disconnect the monitor to eliminate the risk of electric arcing.

ACLS guidelines indicate the medications to be given during cardiac arrest. Although there is limited evidence as to their effectiveness, they should still be given in pregnancy as in any patient experiencing an arrest. The doses do not change.

When a patient is in cardiac arrest, the initial management goals are resuscitation and identifying and aggressively treating reversible causes of the arrest. Several mnemonics have been designed to help with that assessment (**Table 3**). However, it may be more helpful to think of three main categories: (1) hypovolemia, (2) pump failure, and (3) obstruction. Hypovolemia can be caused by massive hemorrhage (external and internal, as from disseminated intravascular coagulation or placental abruption or previa) or vasodilation (septic shock, thyroid storm). Pump failure can result from cardiomyopathy, AMI, or arrhythmia. Obstruction can be the result of pulmonary embolus or pericardial tamponade. Ultrasound can be very useful in assessing these categories. The traditional focused assessment with sonography for trauma examination can diagnose free fluid or pericardial effusion. The subcostal view may be problematic because of the gravid uterus, but other cardiac views (eg, the apical or parasternal long/short) can be helpful to estimate ejection fraction or evaluate for pericardial effusion, right ventricular outflow obstruction, and coordinated cardiac motion. If lack of coordinated cardiac motion is observed or if the mother does not respond to intervention and lacks return of spontaneous circulation, perimortem cesarean section must be considered immediately.

Perimortem cesarean section is a daunting procedure, but one that can be lifesaving for mother and baby. Any pregnant patient with a fundal height at the level of the umbilicus (20 weeks) may benefit from perimortem cesarean section, regardless of fetal viability. One case series reported that 12 of 20 women had return of spontaneous circulation immediately after delivery.[48] Hospitals should have a protocol in place to activate all necessary resources for an emergency cesarean section. Cardiac arrest in a pregnant patient should prompt immediate activation of that protocol (Class I, LOE B recommendation). Cesarean section should be started at 4 minutes after onset of maternal cardiac arrest (Class IIb, LOE C recommendation). Although maternal and fetal outcomes are best when the cesarean section is performed within that window, maternal survival has been reported up to 15 minutes after the onset of arrest, and neonatal survival up to 30 minutes after the onset of arrest. If there is an obvious nonsurvivable maternal injury, or if resuscitation seems futile, it may be appropriate to perform the section immediately, particularly if the fetus is viable.[1]

Table 3	
Reversible causes of cardiac arrest in pregnancy	
Hs & Ts	**BEAU CHOPS**
Hypovolemia	Bleeding/DIC
Hypoxia	Embolism
Hydrogen ions (acidosis)	Anesthetic complications
Hyper/hypokalemia	Uterine atony
Hypothermia	Cardiac disease
Hyper/hypoglycemia	Hypertension/eclampsia
Tablets/toxins	Other
Cardiac tamponade	Placental abruption/previa
Tension pneumothorax	Sepsis
Thrombosis (MI)	
Thromboembolism (PE)	
Trauma	

Abbreviations: DIC, disseminated intravascular coagulation; MI, myocardial infarction; PE, pulmonary embolism.

Data from 2005 American Heart Association Guidelines for Cardiopulmonary Resuscitation and Emergency Cardiovascular Care - Part 7.2: management of cardiac arrest. Circulation 2005;112: IV-58–IV-66.

Therapeutic hypothermia is quickly becoming the standard of care for postarrest nonpregnant patients. Its use in pregnancy is essentially unstudied. One case report documented favorable maternal and fetal outcomes after a term delivery in a patient who suffered arrest early in her pregnancy.[49] The use of therapeutic hypothermia is reasonable to consider, using the same criteria as for nonpregnant patients (Class IIB, LOE C recommendation). Fetal bradycardia is a potential complication, so monitoring is recommended (Class I, LOE C recommendation).[1]

SUMMARY

Cardiovascular emergencies are rare in pregnancy, but when they occur, they are frightening for the patient and the provider. Caring for the critically ill pregnant patient can be quite anxiety provoking, and it is helpful to take a step back and remember that survival of the fetus depends on the health of the mother. Although there are important subtle differences in the treatment of conditions, such as pulmonary embolus, decompensated heart failure, and AMI, the diagnosis and overall goals of management remain the same. Involve consultants early and intervene aggressively but appropriately.

REFERENCES

1. Vanden Hoek T, Morrison LJ. Part 12: Cardiac arrest in special situations. 2010 American Heart Association Guidelines for Cardiopulmonary Resuscitation and Emergency Cardiovascular Care Science. Circulation 2010;122:S829–61.
2. Lewis G, editor. The Confidential Enquiry into Maternal and Child health (CEMACH). Saving mother's lives: reviewing maternal deaths to make motherhood safer—2003–2005. The Seventh report on Confidential Enquiries into Maternal Deaths in the United Kingdom. London: CEMACH; 2007.
3. Dijkman A, Huisman CM, Smit M, et al. Cardiac arrest in pregnancy: increasing use of perimortem caesarean section due to emergency skills training? BJOG 2010;117:282–7.
4. Kline JA, Williams GW, Hernandez-Nino J. D-dimer concentrations in normal pregnancy: new diagnostic thresholds are needed. Clin Chem 2005;51:825–9.
5. Chan WS, Chunilal S, Lee A, et al. A red blood cell agglutination D-dimer test to exclude deep venous thrombosis in pregnancy. Ann Intern Med 2007;147: 165–70.
6. Chan WS, Lee A, Spencer FA, et al. D-dimer testing in pregnant patients: towards determining the next 'level' in the diagnosis of deep vein thrombosis. J Thromb Haemost 2010;8:1004–11.
7. Winer-Muram HT, Boone JM, Brown HL, et al. Pulmonary embolism in pregnant patients: fetal radiation dose with helical CT. Radiology 2002;224:487–92.
8. Department of Health, Government of Western Australia. Diagnostic imaging pathways, March 2012. Available at: www.imagingpathways.health.wa.gov.au/includes/pdf/pe.pdf. Accessed May 3, 2012.
9. Shahir K, Goodman LR, Tali A, et al. Pulmonary embolism in pregnancy: CT pulmonary angiography versus perfusion scanning. Am J Roentgenol 2010; 195(3):W214–20.
10. van Beek EJ, Wild JM, Fink C, et al. MRI for the diagnosis of pulmonary embolism. J Magn Reson Imaging 2003;18:627–40.
11. Duncan KR. The development of magnetic resonance imaging in obstetrics. Br J Hosp Med 1996;55:178–81.
12. Kirkinen P, Partanen K, Vainio P, et al. MRI in obstetrics: a supplementary method for ultrasonography. Ann Med 1996;28:131–6.

13. Turrentine MA, Braems G, Ramirez MM. Use of thrombolytics for the treatment of thromboembolic disease during pregnancy. Obstet Gynecol Surv 1995;50: 534–41.

14. Thabut G, Thabut D, Myers RP, et al. Thrombolytic therapy of pulmonary embolism: a meta-analysis. J Am Coll Cardiol 2002;40:1660–7.

15. Patel RK, Fasan O, Arya R. Thrombolysis in pregnancy. Thromb Haemost 2003; 90:1216–7.

16. Dapprich M, Boessenecker W. Fibrinolysis with alteplase in a pregnant woman with stroke. Cerebrovasc Dis 2002;13:290.

17. Lederer W, Lichtenberger C, Pechlaner C, et al. Long-term survival and neurological outcome of patients who received recombinant tissue plasminogen activator during out-of-hospital cardiac arrest. Resuscitation 2004;61:123–9.

18. Zahorec R. Rescue systemic thrombolysis during cardiopulmonary resuscitation. Bratisl Lek Listy 2002;103:266–9.

19. Li X, Fu QL, Jing XL, et al. A meta-analysis of cardiopulmonary resuscitation with and without the administration of thrombolytic agents. Resuscitation 2006;70: 31–6.

20. DeSanctis RW, Doroghazi RM, Austen WG, et al. Aortic dissection. N Engl J Med 1987;317:1060–7.

21. Mather PJ, Hansen CL, Goldman B, et al. Postpartum multivessel coronary dissection. J Heart Lung Transplant 1994;13:533–7.

22. Immer FF, Bansi AG, Immer-Bansi AS, et al. Aortic dissection in pregnancy: analysis of risk factors and outcome. Ann Thorac Surg 2003;76:309–14.

23. Siu SC, Sermer M, Colman JM, et al. Prospective multicenter study of pregnancy outcomes in women with heart disease. Circulation 2001;104:515–21.

24. Hameed A, Karaalp IS, Tummala PP, et al. The effect of valvular heart disease on maternal and fetal outcome of pregnancy. J Am Coll Cardiol 2001;37:893–9.

25. Campuzano K, Roqué H, Bolnick A, et al. Bacterial endocarditis complicating pregnancy: case report and systematic review of the literature. Arch Gynecol Obstet 2003;268(4):251–5.

26. Siu SC, Sermer M, Harrison DA, et al. Risk and predictors for pregnancy-related complications in women with heart disease. Circulation 1997;96(9):2789–94.

27. Grewal J, Siu SC, Ross HJ, et al. Pregnancy outcomes in women with dilated cardiomyopathy. J Am Coll Cardiol 2009;55:45–52.

28. Cleveland Clinic. B-type natriuretic peptide (BNP) blood test. Available at: http://my.clevelandclinic.org/heart/services/tests/labtests/bnp.aspx. Accessed May 7, 2012.

29. Hameed AB, Chan K, Ghamsary M, et al. Longitudinal changes in the B-type natriuretic peptide levels in normal pregnancy and postpartum. Clin Cardiol 2009;32(8):E60–2.

30. Tanous D, Siu SC, Mason J, et al. B-type natriuretic peptide in pregnant women with heart disease. J Am Coll Cardiol 2010;56:1247–53.

31. James AH, Jamison MG, Biswas MS, et al. Acute myocardial infarction in pregnancy: a United States population-based study. Circulation 2006;113:1564–71.

32. Antman EM, Anbe DT, Armstrong PW, et al. ACC/AHA guidelines for the management of patients with ST-elevation myocardial infarction. Available at: http://assets.cardiosource.com/STEMI_2004.pdf. Accessed May 7, 2012.

33. Low dose aspirin in pregnancy and early childhood development: follow up of the collaborative low dose aspirin study in pregnancy. CLASP collaborative group. Br J Obstet Gynaecol 1995;102:861–8.

34. Hauth JC, Goldenberg RL, Parker CR Jr, et al. Low-dose aspirin: lack of association with an increase in abruptio placentae or perinatal mortality. Obstet Gynecol 1995;85:1055–8.
35. Rubin PC. Current concepts: beta-blockers in pregnancy. N Engl J Med 1981; 305:1323–6.
36. Butters L, Kennedy S, Rubin PC. Atenolol in essential hypertension during pregnancy. BMJ 1990;301:587–9.
37. Lees CC, Lojacono A, Thompson C, et al. Glyceryl trinitrate and ritodrine in tocolysis: an international multicenter randomized study. GTN Preterm Labour Investigation Group. Obstet Gynecol 1999;94:403–8.
38. Gibson PS, Powrie R. Anticoagulants and pregnancy: when are they safe? Cleve Clin J Med 2009;76(2):113–27.
39. Henck JW, Craft WR, Black A, et al. Pre- and postnatal toxicity of the HMG-CoA reductase inhibitor atorvastatin in rats. Toxicol Sci 1998;41:88–99.
40. Drenthen W, Pieper PG, Roos-Hesselink J, et al. Outcome of pregnancy in women with congenital heart disease: a literature review. J Am Coll Cardiol 2007;49(24): 2303–11.
41. Blomström-Lundqvist C, Scheinman MM, Aliot EM, et al. ACC/AHA/ESC guidelines for the management of patients with supraventricular arrhythmias–executive summary: a report of the American College of Cardiology/American Heart Association Task Force on Practice Guidelines and the European Society of Cardiology Committee for Practice Guidelines (Writing Committee to Develop Guidelines for the Management of Patients With Supraventricular Arrhythmias). Circulation 2003;108:1871–909.
42. Cox JL, Gardner MJ. Treatment of cardiac arrhythmias during pregnancy. Prog Cardiovasc Dis 1993;36(2):137–78.
43. Vogel JH, Pryor R, Blount SG Jr. Direct-current defibrillation during pregnancy. JAMA 1965;193:970–1.
44. Page RL. Treatment of arrhythmias during pregnancy. Am Heart J 1995;130(4): 871–6.
45. Barnes EJ, Eben F, Patterson D. Direct current cardioversion during pregnancy should be performed with facilities available for fetal monitoring and emergency caesarean section. BJOG 2002;109(12):1406–7.
46. Dalvi BV, Chaudhuri A, Kulkarni HL, et al. Therapeutic guidelines for congenital complete heart block presenting in pregnancy. Obstet Gynecol 1992;79:802–4.
47. Travers AH, Rea TD, Bobrow BJ, et al. Part 4: CPR overview. 2010 American Heart Association Guidelines for Cardiopulmonary Resuscitation and Emergency Cardiovascular Care. Circulation 2010;122:S676–84.
48. Katz V, Balderston K, DeFreest M. Perimortem cesarean delivery: were our assumptions correct? Am J Obstet Gynecol 2005;192:1916–20.
49. Rittenberger JC, Kelly E, Jang D, et al. Successful outcome utilizing hypothermia after cardiac arrest in pregnancy: a case report. Crit Care Med 2008;36:1354–6.
50. Magee LA, Downar E, Sermer M, et al. Pregnancy outcome after gestational exposure to amiodarone in Canada. Am J Obstet Gynecol 1995;172(4 Pt 1): 1307–11.
51. Magee LA, Schick B, Donnenfeld AE, et al. The safety of calcium channel blockers in human pregnancy: a prospective, multicenter cohort study. Am J Obstet Gynecol 1996;174(3):823–8.
52. Egan DJ, Bisanzo MC, Hutson HR. Emergency department evaluation and management of peripartum cardiomyopathy. J Emerg Med 2009;36:141–7.

Precipitous and Difficult Deliveries

David W. Silver, MD, MA[a,b,*], Frank Sabatino, MD[a,b]

KEYWORDS

- Precipitous delivery • Nuchal cord • Shoulder dystocia • Breech birth
- McRoberts maneuver • Rubin I maneuver • Rotational maneuvers • Frank breech

KEY POINTS

- Emergency deliveries are stressful; have delivery kits prepared as well as protocols for obtaining rapid obstetric and neonatal assistance.
- Check for nuchal cord after delivery of the head.
- More than half of shoulder dystocias can be reduced by using a combination of the McRoberts maneuver and suprapubic pressure.
- Breech delivery should occur by cesarean delivery or in an arena where conversion to cesarean delivery is possible. If vaginal breach delivery occurs, keep hands off of the fetus until the umbilicus is delivered.

A delivery in the emergency department is always a stress-inducing event. The emergency physician must always be ready to assist in a delivery. Although most deliveries are uneventful, several complications need to be resolved quickly to prevent severe morbidity and mortality. Three of the most feared birth complications are nuchal cord, shoulder dystocia, and breech presentation. This article addresses the incidence and maneuvers that can prepare you for these situations and make them less stressful and more successful.

PRECIPITOUS DELIVERY

By definition, any delivery that occurs in the emergency department is precipitous. For many emergency physicians, the initial reaction is to ask how fast the patient can be taken to the labor and delivery (L&D) unit. However, this is not always a feasible option

Funding sources: None.
Conflict of interest: None.
[a] Hofstra North Shore – LIJ School of Medicine, Hempstead, NY, USA; [b] Department of Emergency Medicine, North Shore University Hospital, 300 Community Drive, Manhasset, NY 11030, USA
* Corresponding author. Department of Emergency Medicine, North Shore University Hospital, 300 Community Drive, Manhasset, NY 11030.
E-mail address: dsilver1@nshs.edu

in emergency departments that do not have obstetric support or if the newborn will be delivered before the mother can be transferred safely.

For thousands of years, vaginal births have proceeded naturally and spontaneously, with the only intervention of catching the baby and clamping and cutting the cord. With this in mind, any woman who comes to the emergency department in active labor must have a sterile vaginal examination performed by the treating physician before any decision is made to transfer her to an L&D unit or to an obstetrics receiving hospital. In the community, any woman who is found to be completely dilated and/or effaced should be allowed to deliver before transfer (because delivery in a moving ambulance is less than ideal if a complication arises). Furthermore, any patient that is crowning needs to be delivered in the emergency department whether or not obstetric services are available.

If delivery is deemed imminent, the emergency physician should prepare for 2 patients, both potentially critically ill. Most emergency departments have a baby warmer and packaged kits ready for delivery. If such a setup is not available, make sure you have a neonatal resuscitation kit with infant-sized endotracheal tubes and intubation blades (although in most scenarios only a warm blanket is necessary). A suction device (preferably a blue suction ball) is necessary. Clamps and a scissor must be available for the umbilical cord.

During delivery itself, gentle pressure is applied to the mother's perineum to ease the pressure of descent of the fetus' head (care must be taken not to arrest or apply too much pressure). Once the head delivers and rotates, a finger should be run around the neck to determine if a nuchal cord is present. If identified, the cord should be gently reduced over the head. If this is unsuccessful, another method is to bring the cord caudally over the shoulders and deliver the baby through the cord and then unwind it after delivery.[1]

If this approach also does not work, a summersault maneuver can be used. In this maneuver, the anterior and posterior shoulders should be delivered (slowly) without manipulation of the cord. Simultaneously, the head of the baby is flexed so that the face is pushed toward the maternal thigh. The head is kept close to the perineum as the rest of the body delivers and summersaults out. Once the newborn is delivered, the umbilical cord can be unwrapped and routine postdelivery care initiated.[1]

If none of these techniques seems feasible and the cord is too tight to be reduced, in extreme circumstances, the cord must be clamped and cut before the rest of delivery. This procedure is considered a last resort and comes with its own complications. Very rarely is a nuchal cord a reason for fetal demise or significant morbidity.[2]

Once the neck has been cleared, gentle downward traction is applied on the infant (with caution not to pull traction on the head/neck). Once the anterior shoulder delivers, an upward motion is performed to deliver the posterior shoulder and the rest of the body.

After delivery, the emergency physician must attend to the infant. The mouth and nose should be suctioned. If the baby is not immediately crying, he or she should be stimulated vigorously with a warm blanket. If this does not start spontaneous respirations, bag value masking with positive pressure should be initiated. A pulse should then be sought. If the pulse is less than 60 beats per minute or not present at all, cardiopulmonary resuscitation (CPR) should be started and neonatal resuscitation guidelines should be followed according to the most recent Pediatric Advanced Life Support guidelines (details are beyond the scope of this article).

If circumstances permit, the Apgar score should be calculated. This score is similar to the Glasgow Coma Scale score. It allows easy communication of a baby's status between providers and indicates a basic prognosis for a newborn and is obtained at 1 minutes and 5 minutes after birth. The following mnemonic can be used to remember the categories:

A: Appearance (0: pale or blue, 1: pink body blue extremities, 2: pink body and extremities)

P: Pulse (0: absent, 1: less than 100 beats per minute, 2: more than 100 beats per minute)

G: Grimace (0: absent, 1: grimace or notable facial movement, 2: cough, sneezes, or pulls away)

A: Activity (0: absent, 1: some flexion of extremities, 2: active and spontaneous movements of limbs)

R: Respiration (0: absent, 1: slow and irregular, 2: good breathing with crying)

Each is scored on a scale from 0 to 2. The Apgar score can often be calculated after the delivery and resuscitation is complete as long as the emergency physician keeps in mind what the basic categories are.[3]

To this point, this review discusses the routine parts of a vaginal delivery. The remainder of this article addresses 2 serious complications that require swift and definitive action by the physician to prevent significant morbidity and mortality.

SHOULDER DYSTOCIA

Shoulder dystocia occurs when the anterior shoulder of the infant cannot be delivered under the pubic symphysis. There are no concrete criteria for the diagnosis. One definition encompasses the need for "additional obstetric maneuvers following failure of gentle downward traction on the fetal head to effect delivery of the shoulders."[4] Another focuses on "prolonged head-to-body delivery time (eg, >60 seconds) and/or necessitated use of ancillary obstetric maneuvers."[5] Whichever definition is chosen, the occurrence of shoulder dystocia is a critical time for infant, mother, and emergency physician.

Epidemiology and Risk Factors

Because of the lack of specific criteria, studies examining the prevalence of this type of presentation are limited. The best estimates of the percentage of cases are between 0.2% and 3.0%.[4,6] Several studies demonstrated that Caucasian women and Hispanic women have a lower rate than other racial groups.[7–9] Several other risk factors have also been associated with shoulder dystocia; however, many of them may be unknown to the emergency physician at the time of presentation. The presence of one or multiple risk factors has a poor predicative value for any individual delivery[6,10] and, as discussed later, only suggests that shoulder dystocia may occur. Caution is warranted because preemptive maneuvers are not necessary and can be harmful to the mother.[11]

Risk factors are multifactorial and include maternal, fetal, and intrapartum causes. From a maternal standpoint, gestational or other forms of diabetes, a history of shoulder dystocia, advanced maternal age, postdate pregnancies, obesity, and short stature have all been indicated.[12–14] The only true fetal factor is macrosomia (weight >4000 or 4500 g).[15] A secondary fetal risk factor is male gender.[10,16,17] From an intrapartum standpoint, the risk factor most relevant to the emergency physician is a precipitous delivery.[18,19] This idea seems counterintuitive but it suggests that the fetus does not have the appropriate amount of time to maneuver and rotate into the oblique position in the pelvis, thus keeping shoulders in the wrong orientation at the pelvic brim.[18,20]

Complications

The complications from shoulder dystocia pose dangers to both the mother and the fetus. With regard to the mother, the biggest concerns are postpartum hemorrhage (11%), uterine rupture, and third- and fourth-degree vaginal lacerations (3.8%).[21,22] These types of lacerations lead to higher risks for rectovaginal fistulas and stool incontinence.[13,23]

The consequences to the fetus can be much more serious, causing some of the most litigated complications of birth.[24] The most common injury to the fetus is brachial plexus injury.[25] Excessive traction at the time of delivery can lead to this injury even in the absence of dystocia.[26] This injury can and will occur regardless of the number and type of maneuvers used and is not always the fault of the provider.[27,28] Most brachial plexus injuries are apparent shortly after birth and many, but not all, will resolve by 1 year of age. A specific discussion of the types of brachial plexus injuries is beyond the scope of this article.

Other possible consequences to the fetus are fractures of the clavicle (intentional or unintentional) and the humerus. These fractures occur in approximately 3.0% to 9.5% of shoulder dystocia deliveries.[29,30] Almost all will heal with conservative treatment without any permanent sequelae.[31]

The most devastating complication is hypoxic-ischemic encephalopathy and death. This occurrence is rare and purportedly the result of compression of the umbilical cord, compression of the carotid arteries, and premature separation of the placenta. Studies have demonstrated a linear decline in cord arterial pH with increasing time to delivery.[32,33] The rate of hypoxic encephalopathy and death is very low when the head-to-body delivery time is held to less than 5 minutes.[34]

Management

It is impossible to predict which deliveries will be complicated by shoulder dystocia. Therefore, the provider needs to always be prepared for it. One of the signs to look for early in the delivery is the turtle sign, which is when the fetal head retracts tightly to the mother's perineum and immediately after its presentation.[18] Another common sign is facial flushing as the fetus presents its head. The most reliable finding is that gentle downward traction after presentation of the head fails to deliver the anterior shoulder.

Because shoulder dystocia is unpredictable and uncommon and requires fast and definitive action by the physician, a rational and easy approach is needed. Two commonly used mnemonics are ALARMER and HELPERR (**Fig. 1**).[13] These sequences address the maneuvers that an emergency physician can perform, from least to most invasive. Other more aggressive and invasive procedures are used by obstetricians: the Zavanelli maneuver (cephalic replacement of the head and delaying further contractions to allow for cesarean delivery); clavicle fracture (intentionally breaking the fetal clavicle with manual pressure or an instrument)[35]; symphysiotomy (incision and pressure to open the pubic symphysis to allow passage of the fetus)[36]; and hysterotomy or abdominal rescue (an upper-segment uterine incision that allows the application of more direct pressure or facilitating cephalic replacement).[35]

Maneuvers

When shoulder dystocia is expected, the first step is to always ask for help, that is, mobilize additional resources. Depending on institutional capabilities, requesting assistance from other emergency physicians, obstetricians, pediatricians, operating room staff, anesthesiologists, as well as additional nursing staff is a prudent first step should

ALARMER	HELPERR
A – Ask for Help	H – Help (Call for Help)
L – Leg Hyperflexion (McRoberts')	E – Evaluate for Episiotomy
A – Anterior Shoulder Disimpaction (Suprapubic Pressure or Rubin I)	L – Legs (McRoberts)
R – Rotational Maneuvers (Rubin II or Woods Corkscrew)	P – Pressure (Suprapubic or Rubin I)
M – Manual Delivery of Posterior Arm	E – Entry Maneuvers (Rubin II or Woods Corkscrew)
E – Evaluate for Episiotomy	R – Remove Posterior Arm
R – Roll on all Fours	R – Roll on all Fours

Fig. 1. Two common mnemonics to the approach of a shoulder dystocia.

initial maneuvers not work or the baby and mother both need significant resuscitations. Once someone has been assigned the task of requesting assistance, the following maneuvers can be initiated (presented in the order of least to most invasive).

McRoberts maneuver

According to the American Congress of Obstetricians and Gynecologists, the McRoberts maneuver is a reasonable first strategy.[4] In this procedure, the mother's hips are placed in hyperflexion against the abdomen while being slightly abducted and externally rotated (**Fig. 2**). This position is typically augmented by 2 nurses, each of them holding one of the patient's legs.

The McRoberts maneuver straightens the lumbosacral angle while rotating the symphysis pubis superiorly, which rotates the pelvis over the impacted shoulder, thus freeing it by opening the angle between the sacrum and lumbar spine (**Fig. 3**).[37]

This maneuver alone is successful in reducing up to 40% of cases of dystocia.[6,21,29,30] A meta-analysis revealed that the use of this maneuver does not change the rate of brachial plexus injuries,[38] probably because the delivering physician applies varying amounts of traction.[27] There is no advantage to preemptively instituting the McRoberts positioning to prevent shoulder dystocia.[39,40] To prevent the complications of pubis symphysis damage and femoral neuropathies, prolonged and overaggressive flexion should be avoided.[41]

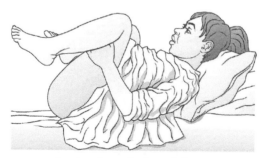

Fig. 2. McRoberts maneuver involves hyperflexion of the mother's hips to the abdomen, with associated external rotation and slight abduction of the legs. (*From* Gottlieb A, Galan H. Shoulder dystocia: an update. Obstet Gynecol Clin North Am 2007;26(2):501–31; with permission.)

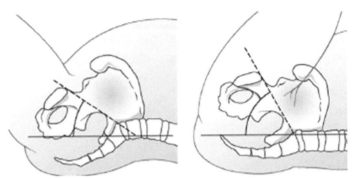

Fig. 3. McRoberts maneuver reorients the maternal pelvis, allowing the shoulders to disimpact from the symphysis pubis. (*From* Gottlieb A, Galan H. Shoulder dystocia: an update. Obstet Gynecol Clin North Am 2007;26(2):501–31; with permission.)

Rubin I maneuver

The Rubin I maneuver has many names, including suprapubic pressure and anterior shoulder disimpaction. In this procedure, downward pressure is applied just proximal to the symphysis pubis by a health care provider who is positioned above the patient to provide better leverage (**Fig. 4**). The pressure can be applied continuously or in a rocking motion (similar to CPR). The pressure being applied adducts the shoulders of the fetus and disimpacts it from the pubic symphysis into an oblique position. Combining this maneuver with the McRoberts maneuver increases the success rate of disimpaction from 40% to nearly 54%.[6]

It is very important to distinguish suprapubic pressure from fundal pressure. Fundal pressure is applied more proximally over the gravid uterus. This fundal pressure would

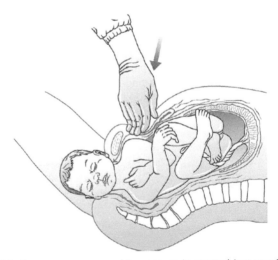

Fig. 4. In the Rubin I maneuver, suprapubic pressure is exerted just proximal to the pubic symphysis onto the fetus' anterior shoulder (*arrow*), with the intent to free it from impaction. Steady constant pressure or a rocking CPR-like motion accomplishes this. (*From* Gottlieb A, Galan H. Shoulder dystocia: an update. Obstet Gynecol Clin North Am 2007;26(2):501–31; with permission.)

in fact worsen the shoulder impaction by rotating the fetus's upper torso against the pubic symphysis.

Rotational maneuvers

Several rotational maneuvers require that the physician's hands enter the vagina and manually attempt to rotate the fetal shoulders to allow disimpaction and delivery. These interventions can be difficult because of the limited space for the clinician's hands to maneuver inside the vagina. If this type of intervention is deemed appropriate, an episiotomy might be necessary (discussed in the next section).

The first of the rotational maneuvers is the Woods screw maneuver. In this procedure, the practitioner inserts his or her hands into the vagina and applies pressure to the anterior aspect of the posterior shoulder, which will abduct/extend the posterior shoulder, rotating the shoulder girdle and freeing it from the pubic symphysis (**Fig. 5**).

The second rotational maneuver is the Rubin II. In this scenario, the practitioner applies pressure to the posterior aspect of the anterior shoulder. This pressure adducts/flexes the anterior shoulder, again changing the orientation of the girdle, freeing it and allowing delivery (**Fig. 6**).

In some circumstances, both maneuvers are used at the same time. However, this approach is most often limited by the amount of room inside the vagina and requires an episiotomy. These procedures can be done with the patient in McRoberts position, enhancing the likelihood of success.

If the two rotational maneuvers discussed earlier fail, one more manipulation can be attempted. In the Reverse Woods Corkscrew, the practitioner places a hand inside the vagina and places it behind the posterior shoulder to flex/abduct it, in essence rotating the fetus in the opposite direction of the previous two maneuvers.

Studies have shown success of up to 60% to 70% with the use of these rotational maneuvers.[40]

Manual delivery of the posterior arm

One of the most effective yet complicated methods of relieving shoulder dystocia is the delivery of the posterior arm. This method has been shown to be effective in up to 84% of situations in which the McRoberts and suprapubic pressure methods have failed.[40] Once again, this is a procedure that requires room within the vaginal vault and could require an episiotomy. The provider must insert his or her hand into the vagina and flex the posterior arm of the fetus, bringing it across the chest. This procedure is best done by finding the antecubital fossa and exerting pressure there. The posterior arm is then delivered over the perineum, which allows the provider to rotate the fetus to allow delivery of the anterior shoulder once the rotation has disimpacted it from the pubic symphysis (**Fig. 7**). Because of its high success rate, some investigators are starting to recommend that it be considered earlier in the delivery algorithm.[39]

One pitfall to be avoided is grasping the upper portion of the posterior arm and exerting traction. This motion can fracture the humerus[42]; but, as mentioned earlier, the resulting injury does not usually lead to long-term morbidity and mortality.

Episiotomy

An episiotomy is an elective incision to widen the perineal area. Shoulder dystocia is an obstruction of bone against bone and not soft tissue.[4] Thus, routine episiotomy is not recommended because it causes perineal trauma without providing much benefit in terms of relieving neonatal distress and risking brachial plexus injuries.[43,44] However, in extreme cases, episiotomy becomes necessary to provide space for rotational maneuvers and posterior arm deliveries undertaken to prevent permanent hypoxic injury to the fetus.

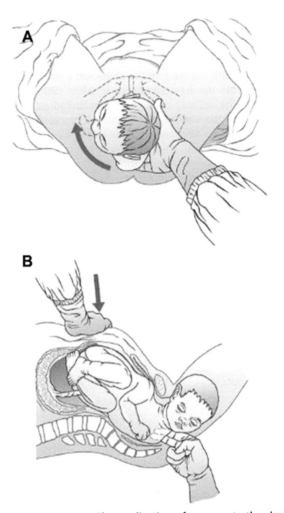

Fig. 5. Woods corkscrew maneuver. The application of pressure to the clavicular surface of the posterior arm allows rotation, dislodging the anterior shoulder from behind the maternal symphysis. (*A*) Curved arrow illustrates rotation. (*B*) Straight arrow shows manual rotation of infant's body while rotation is in progress. (*From* Gottlieb A, Galan H. Shoulder dystocia: an update. Obstet Gynecol Clin North Am 2007;26(2):501–31; with permission.)

Two types of episiotomies are performed: median and mediolateral. In the median approach, an incision is made at the posterior fourchette and extended 2.5 cm in the midline posteriorly. If time permits, anesthesia induced by lidocaine is preferred but is often not possible in this type of scenario. In the mediolateral approach, an incision is made from the midpoint of the fourchette and extended to the right or left 2.5 cm, which runs in a diagonal line from the anus (midpoint between the anus and the ischial tuberosity). A scalpel or Metzenbaum scissors can be used for this procedure.

Gaskin position

The Gaskin position (or *roll on all fours*) is an effective technique that can be performed quickly and safely to help resolve shoulder dystocia.[45] Simply placing the mother in a hands-and-knees position (**Fig. 8**) can facilitate a spontaneous delivery. In one

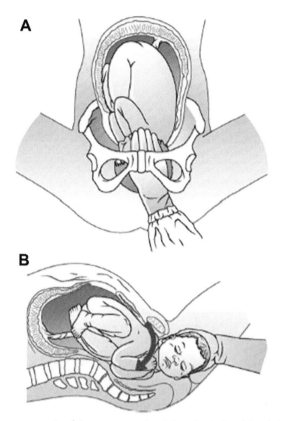

Fig. 6. Rubin II maneuver. Applying pressure to either fetal shoulder (whichever is more accessible, anterior or posterior) to effect shoulder adduction (*A*). Curved arrow shows rotation of fetal shoulders (*B*). (*From* Gottlieb A, Galan H. Shoulder dystocia: an update. Obstet Gynecol Clin North Am 2007;26(2):501–31; with permission.)

study, 83% of women who were moved into this position delivered without any further maneuvers needed.[45] This positioning initially may be disorienting to the physician; but it allows gravity and increased space near the sacrum to deliver the posterior shoulder and arm, thus disimpacting the anterior shoulder from the pubic symphysis.[46]

BREECH PRESENTATION

As previously stated, the emergency department is a suboptimal place for delivery.[47] In virtually all circumstances, the mother should be transferred to an L&D unit where cesarean delivery can be performed, if necessary.[48,49] Controversy remains regarding the most successful delivery options for a term breech presentation. Most investigators recommend cesarean delivery.[48–51] Circumstances, such as precipitous delivery, lack of prenatal care, and the mother's preference for vaginal delivery, can place an emergency medicine physician in the situation of managing a breech delivery. This discussion is especially relevant to the emergency department scenarios in which vaginal delivery is imminent without obstetric backup or if the physician is concerned about fetal demise.

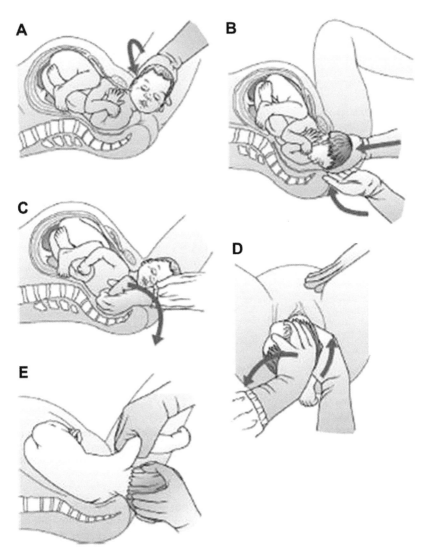

Fig. 7. Delivery of the posterior shoulder. For delivery of the posterior arm, to flex the fetal foreman, apply pressure at the antecubital fossa. While holding the forearm or hand, move the arm over the infant's chest and deliver over the perineum. It may be necessary to rotate the trunk to move the posterior arm anteriorly. (*A*) Turn the fetal head to make room for the practitioner's hand. (*B*) Hold fetal head with one hand while moving the second hand posteriorly. (*C*) To grasp the posterior forearm or hand, flex the infant's arm at the antecubital fossa. (*D*) Posterior arm is delivered. (*E*) For delivery, continue rotating the fetus. (*From* Gottlieb A, Galan H. Shoulder dystocia: an update. Obstet Gynecol Clin North Am 2007;26(2):501–31; with permission.)

Breech presentations occur in 3% to 4% of term pregnancies.[52] They are associated with a morbidity rate 3 to 4 times greater than that of normal cephalad presentations.[51,52] Breech presentations occur more frequently with premature infants because the final natural rotation in the pelvis may not have occurred.

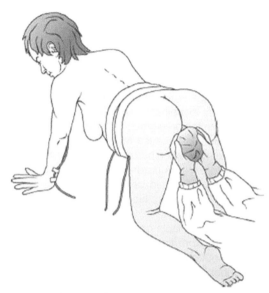

Fig. 8. The Gaskin maneuver is accomplished by placing the patient on all fours. This potentiates delivery of the posterior shoulder using gravity and increased dimensions of the maternal pelvis. (*From* Gottlieb A, Galan H. Shoulder dystocia: an update. Obstet Gynecol Clin North Am 2007;26(2):501–31; with permission.)

Breech presentation is associated with a greater incidence of fetal distress and umbilical cord prolapse, but the feared complication of breech deliveries is head entrapment, which can lead to asphyxiation and death.[51] In a normal cephalic presentation, the head maximally dilates the birth canal, allowing the rest of the body to descend unobstructed. However, with a breech presentation, the head emerges last and can be entrapped by incomplete cervical dilation.[51]

Breech presentations are classified based on presenting position: frank, complete, incomplete, or footling. In frank breech, the most common, the baby's buttocks are first into the birth canal, the hips are flexed, and the knees are extended with the feet adjacent to the head. Up to 65% to 70% of breech positions are in frank position. In complete breech, the baby again presents with the buttocks first, but both the hips and knees are flexed. The baby might sit cross-legged. With frank or complete breech, the buttocks can act as a wedge that dilates the cervix, allowing the delivery to proceed in an uncomplicated way.[51] In incomplete or footling breech, one or both of the baby's feet lie below the breech, so the foot or knee is the first presenting part into the birth canal. Incomplete or footling breech positions are rare overall but more common with premature fetuses.

Management

The first step for an emergency physician confronted with a fetus in breech presentation is to obtain obstetric consultation immediately. Additionally, the emergency physician should obtain the help of several assistants. One crucial point to remember when attempting vaginal delivery of a breech position is to minimize touching the fetus and let the delivery happen spontaneously. The rationale is that the presenting part will maximize the dilation of the birth canal. In fact, it is recommended that the fetus not be touched until the umbilicus has presented.[51] A second important point for the delivering examiner is to never pull on the fetus. Excessive traction can extend the fetal head, which leads to entrapment of the head and greatly increases the risk of asphyxiation.

Initial Preparation

If possible, ultrasound imaging should be performed early in labor to determine the fetal position. A sterile vaginal examination should also be performed to assess for position as well as to ascertain the presenting fetal part. The practitioner should avoid premature rupture of membranes because the abnormal breech position increases cord compression. Once the membrane has ruptured during labor, a vaginal examination should be performed to exclude cord prolapse. Additionally, continuous electronic fetal heart rate monitoring should be used because of the increased risk of cord compression.[53] From this point on, labor and monitoring should progress as in a cephalic delivery.

Epidural anesthesia remains a viable option during breech delivery. It can relieve pain and prevent the mother from involuntary pushing before cervical dilatation is maximized. However, the mother needs to be able to push effectively once the breech descends into the pelvic floor.[53] Alternatively, a pudendal block can be used once the fetus has descended to the pelvic floor.[54]

Delivery Technique

When presented with the active delivery of a fetus in breech presentation, the mother should be placed in the lithotomy position. She should be encouraged to bear down until the infant's feet, legs, and trunk are visible. If the feet and legs are not extended, the clinician can let the delivery continue spontaneously with maternal effort. The fetal body should be supported at an angle at or below the angle of the birth canal.[51] The presenting parts should not be raised upward. Again, clinicians should be warned not to apply traction to the fetus.

If the legs and feet are extended, the clinician should perform the Pinard maneuver. The first step of this maneuver is to place a hand behind the fetal thigh and press gently in a lateral direction, allowing delivery of the leg. A similar technique is used to deliver the opposite leg.[51,54]

Maternal expulsion efforts should be significant enough to deliver to the point of the umbilicus. It is important to keep the sacrum of the fetus in the anterior direction. Continue to deliver and support the fetus until the clavicles are delivered, ensuring that the fetal sacrum remains anterior. The next step is to deliver the arms. Rotate the fetus 90° in a counterclockwise direction. If spontaneous delivery of the arms does not occur, one of the examiner's fingers can be placed along the scapula over the shoulder and into the antecubital fossa, where gentle pressure is applied by the flexing the finger, allowing the arm to be delivered.[51,54] To deliver the other arm, rotate the fetus 180° in a counterclockwise direction and use a similar approach. Once both arms have been delivered, the baby is rotated so that the sacrum is anterior again. The next step is delivery of the head.

An assistant should be present to apply strong suprapubic pressure to encourage the head to flex. If the fetal head does not appear spontaneously, the examiner should place his or her right arm under the fetus for support and reach into the birth canal. The clinician's fingers should apply pressure to the maxillary processes of the fetus to achieve flexion of the head.[51] The fetal body should be kept parallel to the floor. Excessive upward angulation and traction will cause hyperextension of the neck and can cause injury to the cervical spinal cord.[47]

Head entrapment is a dangerous complication of breech presentation. If the head becomes entrapped, a uterine relaxant should be administered.[54] Ideally, a β-adrenergic agonist, such as terbutaline, 0.25 mg subcutaneously, 2.5 to 10 μg/min intravenously. Intravenous administration of nitroglycerin, 50 to 200 μg, is an alternative. This dose may promote enough uterine relaxation to promote head delivery.[54]

SUMMARY

Most fetuses in breech presentations are delivered via cesarean delivery. Certain circumstances mandate that emergency physicians be prepared to manage urgent delivery of a breech presentation. On presentation, an obstetrician should be contacted immediately. If delivery is imminent, ultrasound and vaginal examinations should be performed to determine fetal positioning. Anesthesia can be provided via spinal epidural or with a pudendal block. The clinician should allow maternal effort to deliver spontaneously while supporting the fetus. At no time should traction be placed on the fetus. The clinician can aid delivery by performing the Pinard maneuver. If needed, a β-agonist, such as terbutaline or nitroglycerin, can be used to facilitate delivery of the head.

Although rare and often uneventful, precipitous deliveries within the emergency department can be quite chaotic. The fear of complications escalates the intensity of these situations. The 3 most commonly encountered difficulties are nuchal cord, shoulder dystocia, and breech presentation. The basic treatment and interventions for each are reviewed in this article. Keeping a calm mind and a adopting a methodical and stepwise approach will help ensure successful outcomes for precipitous deliveries in the emergency department.

REFERENCES

1. Mercer J, Skovgaard R, Peareara J, et al. Nuchal cord management and nurse-midwifery practice. J Midwifery Womens Health 2005;50:373–9.
2. Rhrestha N, Singh N. Nuchal cord and perinatal outcome. Kathmandu Univ Med J (KUMJ) 2007;5(3):360–3.
3. Casey B, McIntire D, Leveno K. The continuing value of the Apgar score for the assessment of newborn infants. N Engl J Med 2001;344(7):467–71.
4. Gynocologists ACoOa. Shoulder dystocia, ACOG practice bulletin clinical management guidelines for obstretrician-gynocologists. Obstet Gynecol 2002; 100(100):1045–50.
5. Spong C, Beall M, Rodrigues D. An objective definition of shoulder dystocia: prolonged head to body delivery intervals and/or use of ancillary obstetric maneuvers. Obstet Gynecol 1995;86:433–6.
6. Gherman R. Shoulder dystocia: an evidence based evaluation of the obstetric nightmare. Clin Obstet Gynecol 2002;45:345–62.
7. Cheng Y, Norwitz E, Caughey A. The relationship of fetal position and ethnicity with shoulder dystocia and birth injury. Am J Obstet Gynecol 2006;195:856–62.
8. Nesbit T, Gilbert W, Herrchen B. Shoulder dystocia and associated risk factors with macrosomic infants born in California. Am J Obstet Gynecol 1998;179(2): 476–80.
9. Wolf H, Hoeksma A, Oei S. Obstetric brachial plexus injury: risk factors related to recovery. Eur J Obstet Gynecol Reprod Biol 2000;88:133–8.
10. Geary M, McParland P, Johnson H. Shoulder dystocia: is it predictable? Eur J Obstet Gynecol Reprod Biol 1995;62:15–8.

11. Anderson J. Complications of labor and delivery: shoulder dystocia. Prim Care 2012;39:135–44.
12. Baskett T. Shoulder dystocia. Best Pract Res Clin Obstet Gynaecol 2002;16(1): 57–68.
13. Baxlet E, Gobbo R. Shoulder dystocia. Am Fam Physician 2004;69(7):1707–14.
14. Gherman R, Chauhan S, Ouzounian V. Shoulder dystocia: the unpreventable obstetric emergency with empiric management guidelines. Am J Obstet Gynecol 2006;195(3):657–72.
15. Weeks J, Pitman T, Spinnato I. Fetal macrosomia: does antenatal prediction affect delivery route and birth outcome? Am J Obstet Gynecol 1995;173(4):1215–9.
16. Hassaan A. Should dystocia: risk factors and prevention. Aust N Z J Obstet Gynaecol 1988;28:107–9.
17. Mandany AE, Jallard K, Radi F. Shoulder dystocia: anticipation and outcome. Int J Gynaecol Obstet 1990;34:7–12.
18. Gherman R. Shoulder dystocia: prevention and management. Obstet Gynecol Clin North Am 2005;32:297–305.
19. Poggi S, Stallings S, Ghindi A. Intrapartum risk factors for permanent brachial plexus injury. Am J Obstet Gynecol 2003;189:725–9.
20. Gherman R, Goodwin T, Ouzounian J. Brachial plexus palsy associated with cesarean section: an in utero injury? Am J Obstet Gynecol 1997;177(5):1162–4.
21. Gherman R, Goodwin T, Souter I. The McRoberts' maneuver for the alleviation of shoulder dystocia: how successful is it? Am J Obstet Gynecol 1997;176:656–61.
22. Gottlieb A, Galan H. Shoulder dystocia: an update. Obstet Gynecol Clin North Am 2007;26(2):501–31.
23. Wagner R, Nielsen P, Gonik B. Shoulder dystocia. Obstet Gynecol Clin North Am 1999;26(2):371–83.
24. Gilbert W, Nesbit T, Danielsen B. Associated factors in 1611 cases of brachial plexus injury. Obstet Gynecol 1999;93(4):536–40.
25. Doumouchtsis S, Arulkumaran S. Is it possible to reduce obstetrical brachial plexus palsy by optimal management of should dystocia? Ann N Y Acad Sci 2010;1205:135–43.
26. Allen R, Sorab J, Gonik B. Risk factors for shoulder dystocia: an engineering study of clinician applied forces. Obstet Gynecol 1991;77:352–5.
27. Baskett T, Allen A. Perinatal implications of shoulder dystocia. Obstet Gynecol 1995;86:14–7.
28. Nocon J, McKenzie D, Thomas L. Shoulder dystocia: an analysis of risks and obstetric maneuvers. Am J Obstet Gynecol 1993;168:1732–9.
29. Gherman R, Ouzounian J, Goodwin T. Obstetric maneuvers for shoulder dystocia and associated fetal morbidity. Am J Obstet Gynecol 1998;178(6):1126–30.
30. McFarland M, Langer O, Piper J. Perinatal outcome and the type and number of maneuvers in shoulder dystocia. Int J Gynaecol Obstet 1996;55:219–24.
31. Nadas S, Reinberg O. Obstetric fractures. Eur J Pediatr Surg 1992;2:165–8.
32. Leung T, Stuart O, Sahota D. Head-to-body delivery interval and risk of fetal acidosis and hypoxic ischaemic encephalopathy in should dystocia: a retrospective review. BJOG 2011;118(4):474–9.
33. Stallings S, Edwards R, Johnson J. Correlation of head-to-body delivery intervals in should dystocia and umbilical artery acidosis. Am J Obstet Gynecol 2001;185: 268–74.
34. Beer E, Folghera M. Time for resolving shoulder dystocia. Am J Obstet Gynecol 1998;179:1376–7.

35. Kwek K, Yeo G. Shoulder dystocia and injuries: prevention and management. Curr Opin Obstet Gynecol 2006;18:123–8.
36. Goodwin T, Banks E, Lynnae K. Catastrophic shoulder dystocia and emergency symphysiotomy. Am J Obstet Gynecol 1997;177:463–4.
37. Gherman R, Tramont J, Muffley P, et al. Analysis of McRoberts' maneuver by x-ray pelvimetry. Obstet Gynecol 2000;95:43–7.
38. MacKenzie I, Mutayyab S, Lean K. Management of shoulder dystocia: trends in incidence and maternal and neonatal morbidity. Obstet Gynecol 2011;110(5):1059–68.
39. Hoffman M, Bailit J, Branck D, et al. A comparison of obstetric maneuvers for the acute management of shoulder dystocia. Obstet Gynecol 2011;117:1272–8.
40. Leung T, Stuart O, Suen S, et al. Comparison of perinatal outcomes of shoulder dystocia alleviated by different type and sequence of manoeuvers: a retrospective review. BJOG 2011;118:985–90.
41. Gherman R, Ouzounian J, Incerpi M. Symphyseal separation and transient femoral neuropathy associated with McRoberts' maneuver. Am J Obstet Gynecol 1998;178(3):609–10.
42. Thompson K, Satin A, Gherman R. Spiral fracture of the radius: an unusual case of shoulder dystocia-associated morbidity. Obstet Gynecol 2003;102:36–8.
43. Dandolu V, Jain N, Hernandez E. Shoulder dystocia at noninstrumental vaginal delivery. Am J Perinatol 2006;23(7):439–44.
44. Gurewitsch E, Donithan M, Stallings S. Episiotomy versus fetal manipulation in managing severe shoulder dystocia" A comparison of outcomes. Am J Obstet Gynecol 2004;191:911–6.
45. Bruner J, Drummond S, Meenan A, et al. All-fours maneuver for reducing shoulder dystocia during labor. J Reprod Med 1998;43(5):439–43.
46. Kovavisarach E. The "all-fours" maneuver for the management of shoulder dystocia. Int J Gynaecol Obstet 2006;95(2):153–4.
47. Stallard T, Burns B. Emergency delivery and perimortem C-section. Emerg Med Clin North Am 2003;21:679–93.
48. Gynecologists ACoOa. Mode of term singleton breech delivery. Washington DC: American College of Obstetricians and Gynecologists; 2001. Contract No.: committee opinion number 265.
49. Mazhar S, Kausar S. Outcome of singleton breech deliveries beyond 28 weeks gestation: the experience at MCH Centre, PIMS. J Pak Med Assoc 2002;52:471.
50. Gilbert W, Hicks S, Danielsen B. Vaginal versus cesarean delivery for breech presentation in California: a population based study. Obstet Gynecol 2003;102:911–7.
51. Tintinalli J, Kelen G, Stapczynski J, et al. Tintinalli's emergency medicine. 6th edition. New York: McGraw-Hill; 2004.
52. Hearne A, Driggers R. The Johns Hopkins manual of gynecology and obstetrics. 2nd edition. Baltimore (MD): Johns Hopkins University Press; 2002.
53. Kotaska A, Menticoglou S, Gagnon R. Vaginal delivery of Breech Presentation. J Obstet Gynaecol Can 2009;31:557.
54. Shah K, Mason C. Essential emergency procedures. Philadelphia: Lippincott; 2008.

Obstetric Toxicology: Teratogens

Michael Levine, MD[a,b,*], Ayrn D. O'Connor, MD[b]

KEYWORDS

• Antibiotic • Anticoagulant • Antihypertensive • Antiarrhythmic • Anticonvulsant
• Pregnancy • Teratogen • Teratogenicity

KEY POINTS

• The pregnancy risk classification developed by the US Food and Drug Administration is an imperfect source of information and should not be relied on to determine treatment or guide counseling of pregnant patients.

• An accurate, up-to-date, readily available source of information to guide clinicians in determining the teratogenic risks of medications is needed.

• Proper education and counseling of pregnant patients are paramount. Clinicians are encouraged to seek expert advice from teratologists when data regarding an agent's safety are limited or conflicting.

INTRODUCTION

Annually, more than 6.4 million pregnancies occur in the United States, with a resulting 4.14 million live births.[1] Many of the women carrying these pregnancies are treated in US emergency departments (ED). Although the exact prevalence of pregnancy among ED patients is not known, by some estimates nearly 10% of all women seeking care in an ED are pregnant.[2] Consequently, emergency physicians need to be familiar with which drugs should be avoided in pregnancy and which drugs are deemed safe.

An important historical event changed our understanding of pharmaceutical teratogens. In 1956, thalidomide was used for the treatment of influenza.[3] Shortly thereafter, it was used as a sedative and ultimately as an antiemetic during pregnancy. It was marketed under 37 names worldwide, but it never received approval from the US Food and Drug Administration (FDA) because of concerns about its safety.[4,5] When administered to pregnant women, many of their offspring developed a pattern of malformations consisting of phocomelia, thumb aplasia, congenital heart and ear defects,

Disclosures: There are no financial, legal, or other conflicts of interest involved in the preparation of this article.
[a] Section of Medical Toxicology, Department of Emergency Medicine, University of Southern California, 1200 North State Street, Room 1011, Los Angeles, CA 90033, USA; [b] Department of Medical Toxicology, Banner Good Samaritan Medical Center, 925 East McDowell Road, Second Floor, Phoenix, AZ 85006, USA
* Corresponding author. Section of Medical Toxicology, Department of Emergency Medicine, University of Southern California, 1200 North State Street, Room 1011, Los Angeles, CA 90033, USA.
E-mail address: mdlevine@usc.edu

Emerg Med Clin N Am 30 (2012) 977–990
http://dx.doi.org/10.1016/j.emc.2012.08.008
0733-8627/12/$ – see front matter © 2012 Elsevier Inc. All rights reserved.

duodenal atresia, and triphalangism.[4,5] The drug was withdrawn worldwide in the early 1960s after its teratogenic effects were confirmed. Fewer than 30 pharmaceutical agents are proven human teratogens when administered at clinically relevant doses.[6] Of the known teratogens, only a few remain in clinical use (**Table 1**).

Following this important historical event, awareness of the potential teratogenic effects increased, as did regulation. Pharmaceutical manufacturers are required by law to label their products regarding use in pregnancy according to standards established by the FDA. The FDA categorizes prescription drugs according to their risk of causing fetal harm (**Table 2**). This classification is based on the strength of evidence available at the time a drug is approved. Category C is the default category, and most drugs fall into this group. Because the risk is unknown, the drug might be capable of teratogenic effects or it might be perfectly safe. This classification system has many limitations and many teratologists find it misleading. It is often criticized for being overly conservative, it is rarely updated or revised, and medicolegal or liability issues may drive an agent's classification. Consequently, clinicians cannot rely on this categorization as a reliable, updated source of information to guide their practice. And, as in the nonpregnant population, prescription drug use among pregnant women is common. In one Canadian population-based study, 63.5% of pregnant women consumed a prescription medication during their pregnancy, with nearly 8% of these being category D or X medications.[7] In a similar study in the United States involving more than 150 000 births identified through 8 health maintenance organizations, 64% of the women received a prescription medication during their pregnancy and 9.4% of them received a category D or X medication.[8]

Many pharmaceutical agents known to be human teratogens have either been removed from the market or are not likely to be prescribed by emergency physicians (eg, thalidomide, diethylstilbestrol, systemic isotretinoin). Environmental exposures or drugs of abuse (eg, radiation, methylmercury, ethanol) are beyond the scope of this article. Thus, this review focuses on those drugs likely to be prescribed by emergency physicians during their routine practice and care of pregnant patients. In addition, this

Table 1	
Drugs with known teratogenic effects in humans	
Drug	**Clinical Effects**
Methotrexate	CNS and limb malformations
ACE inhibitors	Renal failure, renal dysgenesis, skull malformations
Antithyroid drugs (PTU, methimazole)	Fetal goiter, hypothyroidism
Carbamazepine	Neural tube defects
Lithium	Ebstein anomaly
Misoprostol	Moebius syndrome
Phenytoin	CNS deficits, growth retardation
Retinoids	CNS, craniofacial, CV, and other defects
Tetracycline	Anomalies of the teeth and bone
Thalidomide	Phocomelia
Valproic acid	Neural tube defects
Warfarin	Skeletal and CNS defects, Dandy-Walker syndrome

Abbreviations: ACE, angiotensin-converting enzyme; CNS, central nervous system; CV, cardiovascular; PTU, propylthiouracil.

This table represents known teratogens still clinically available and potentially encountered by emergency physicians. It does not represent an all-encompassing list.

Data from Koren G, Pastuszak A, Ito S. Drugs in pregnancy. N Engl J Med 1998;338:1128–37.

Table 2	
FDA classification of drugs based on pregnancy risk	
Class	**Description**
A	There is no risk. Adequate and well-controlled studies failed to demonstrate fetal risk.
B	There is no evidence suggesting risk. Animal studies failed to demonstrate risk to the fetus and there are no adequate studies in pregnant women.
C	There may be a risk to the fetus. Animal studies have demonstrated an adverse effect on the fetus, but there are no well-performed studies in humans.
D	There is evidence of fetal risk, but there may be situations in which the benefits exceed the real risk.
X	There is evidence of fetal risk. There are no known circumstances under which the benefits exceed the risk.

Data from Addis A, Sharabi S, Bonati M. Risk classification systems for drug use during pregnancy: are they a reliable source of information? Drug Saf 2000;23:245–53.

article discusses potential toxicities from obstetric treatments that may be instituted in the ED.

KNOWN HUMAN TERATOGENS

Anticoagulants

Warfarin is a vitamin K antagonist that has long been used for the management and prophylaxis of venothromboembolic events. Warfarin inhibits vitamin K production by altering the vitamin K cycle through the inhibition of several enzymes, including vitamin K epoxide reductase.

Warfarin interferes with the fetal synthesis of various proteins that are instrumental in bone and cartilage formation. The period of greatest susceptibility to bone and cartilage malformation is during weeks 6 to 12 of gestation.[9] Commonly encountered clinical features of fetuses with in utero exposure to warfarin include shortening/flattening of the nose, laryngomalacia, congenital heart defects (atrial septal defect, patent ductus arteriosus), growth retardation, and telebrachydactyly.[10] Fetal hemorrhage is common and in one case series was present in 8 out of 13 (61.5%) fetuses.[11] The hemorrhages occurred in all trimesters and were typically associated with diffuse hemorrhage. Radiographs can demonstrate bony stippling of the epiphyses.[11,12] Thus, warfarin should be avoided throughout pregnancy. Low-molecular-weight heparin injections are a safe alternative for outpatient therapy.

Anticonvulsants

More than 1.1 million women of childbearing age have epilepsy.[13] Although avoidance of any antiepileptic drug during pregnancy may be ideal in theory, the risk of in utero drug exposure must be weighed against the real risk of seizing, which is also detrimental to the fetus. Strong evidence is lacking, but it is generally thought that there is a greater risk of fetal harm from a seizure than from use of antiepileptic drugs.[14] As a result, optimal management involves using the lowest effective dose of antiepileptic drug as monotherapy whenever possible.[14,15] The pharmacokinetics of many anticonvulsants, such as elimination and volume of distribution, are altered during pregnancy.[14,15] As a result, drug levels should be monitored closely, if possible. If phenobarbital, valproic acid, phenytoin, carbamazepine, or levetiracetam is administered to pregnant patients, drug concentrations should be measured.[15,16] Because primidone is metabolized to phenobarbital, concentrations of that metabolite can be used to monitor therapeutic efficacy.

Carbamazepine

Carbamazepine is commonly used for the management of seizures as well as other conditions, including chronic pain syndromes. A recent meta-analysis examining the teratogenic properties of carbamazepine found a 2.6-fold increased risk of spina bifida compared with controls.[17] The rate of spina bifida with carbamazepine was much lower than with valproic acid, and the rate of cleft lip was lower than that associated with most other anticonvulsant drugs.[17] However, its use in pregnancy should be avoided.

Phenytoin

Phenytoin is used for the management of many primary seizure disorders. In the early 1970s, concern was raised about the possibility of a teratogenic potential of phenytoin.[18] Fetal hydantoin syndrome is a constellation of minor facial abnormalities and terminal digital changes. Digital changes ascribed to fetal hydantoin syndrome include hypoplasia of the fingers and toes, with associated stiffness of the interphalangeal joints. Midface hypoplasia is encountered with approximately the same frequency as digital hypoplasia. Microcephaly and intrauterine growth retardation are rare.[19]

Seven studies examined the teratogenic risk of fetal malformations following intrauterine exposure to phenytoin when used as monotherapy. In these studies, the relative risk for fetal toxicity exceeded 1.0 in 4 out of 7 studies, and in no study was statistical significance achieved.[20] Thus, although phenytoin may have teratogenic effects, the incidence is rare.[20] Nonetheless, given that it is a known teratogen, its administration should be based on an individual approach to patients after weighing the risks and benefits of its use and in consultation with specialists, such as an obstetrician or a neurologist.

Valproic acid

Valproic acid is widely used as an anticonvulsant and a mood stabilizer for various psychiatric disorders. Following its introduction, its teratogenic effects were not immediately recognized. Later, when this potential was observed, it was difficult to fully ascribe the fetal malformations to valproic acid because many cases involved combination therapy with other anticonvulsants.[20] Ultimately, further studies estimated that maternal use of valproic acid during the first trimester is associated with a 7-fold increased risk of the fetus being born with major malformations.[21]

Fetal valproate syndrome involves both minor and major malformations. Of these, craniofacial abnormalities are most common and include epicanthal folds, a flattened nasal bridge with upturned nose, small ears, a long and flat philtrum, and a thin vermilion border.[21,22] Neural tube defects are common. Several mechanisms have been proposed to explain the association between valproic acid and neural tube defects, but no definitive consensus has been reached. Despite not knowing the definitive cause of neural tube defects, the risk is clear; a birth defect surveillance program identified a 20-fold increased risk of spina bifida following in utero exposure to valproic acid.[23]

Fetal cardiac abnormalities are also commonly encountered as part of the fetal valproate syndrome. Ventricular septal defect, aortic stenosis, and pulmonary stenosis are among the most common.[22]

Infants born with fetal valproate syndrome have a higher mortality rate than those without valproate exposure. In one series, 12% of children born with fetal valproate syndrome died during infancy and another 29% had significant developmental delay.[22]

ANTIMETABOLITES

Methotrexate is a folic acid antagonist that is commonly used for the treatment of several rheumatologic and oncologic conditions. Methotrexate inhibits the enzyme dihydrofolate reductase, an enzyme involved in DNA synthesis.[24] Methotrexate embryopathy is characterized by microcephaly, short limbs, growth retardation, hypoplastic skull with wide fontanels, craniosynostosis, and numerous other minor physical anomalies involving facial features. In general, fetal harm is caused by dosages higher than 10 mg/wk.[24]

Emergency physicians occasionally administer methotrexate as a treatment of ectopic pregnancies. The use of methotrexate for medical management of an ectopic pregnancy becomes problematic in cases involving an unrecognized intrauterine or heterotopic pregnancy. In addition to the previously mentioned problems, there is some concern for an increased prevalence of tetralogy of Fallot when methotrexate is used very early in pregnancy, as might occur during the medical management of an ectopic pregnancy.[24–26]

ANTIMICROBIALS

One of the greatest advances in modern medicine is the advent of antimicrobials. Although the appropriate antimicrobial can be life saving in the event of an infection, teratogenic effects must be considered when antimicrobials are administered to pregnant patients. It is important that the emergency physician choose an antimicrobial with the appropriate spectrum of coverage while avoiding unnecessary risk to the fetus.

Tetracyclines

Tetracyclines are broad-spectrum bacteriostatic drugs that inhibit protein synthesis. They are effective against many gram-positive and gram-negative organisms. When administered systemically, they cross the placenta and can result in a yellow-brown discoloration of permanent teeth.[27,28] Topically applied tetracycline, however, is unlikely to be teratogenic because systemic concentrations are rarely elevated enough to cause fetal injury.[29] Oxytetracycline, a specific type of tetracycline, is associated with an increased risk of neural tube defects, cleft palate, and cardiovascular disease. Of note, treatment with a tetracycline derivative, such as doxycycline, is unlikely to be teratogenic; therefore, its use is not thought to be contraindicated.[29,30] As with most drugs, the safest option should always be used, but if doxycycline is thought to be the most appropriate medication for a particular situation, its use is acceptable.[29,31]

In addition to the dental abnormalities associated with tetracycline, the medication is associated with inhibition of calcium uptake and elongation in the long bones. These effects can inhibit bone growth; however, this inhibition is only temporary and is rapidly reversible on discontinuation of the medication.[32]

CARDIOVASCULAR MEDICATIONS
ACE Inhibitors and Angiotensin II Receptor Antagonists

Angiotensin-converting enzyme inhibitors (ACE-I) are commonly used for the management of hypertension as well as renal protection in patients with diabetes. These drugs act as competitive inhibitors of ACE, thereby increasing bradykinin levels and inhibiting the formation of angiotensin II (and subsequently aldosterone). This combination results in increased vasodilation and reduced sodium and water retention.[33] Similarly, angiotensin II receptor antagonists directly decrease aldosterone production.

Traditionally, the use of ACE-I has been considered contraindicated in the second and third trimesters, with fetal exposure during this period resulting in impaired renal formation and function. Consequently, fetal urine production is decreased, causing oligohydramnios and resultant intrauterine growth retardation.[34,35] Additional complications aside from oligohydramnios, which are observed as part of ACE-I fetopathy, include retarded ossification of skull bones, limb deformities, and neonatal renal failure.[35,36] A similar constellation of symptoms has been observed following the administration of angiotensin II receptor antagonists.[37] Cooper and colleagues[38] questioned the timing of exposure versus fetal risk and demonstrated increased relative risk of major congenital malformations following the first-trimester use of ACE-I. Consequently, the use of ACE-I should be avoided throughout the pregnancy. **Table 3** lists the FDA pregnancy categories of several commonly used antihypertensives.

Amiodarone

Amiodarone is a nonselective antidysrhythmic whose primary indication is the management of ventricular dysrhythmias, although it can be used for some supraventricular dysrhythmias.[39] It readily crosses the placenta and, because of its high iodine content, has high affinity for fetal thyroid tissue.[40,41] Amiodarone's effects on the thyroid gland can be divided into iodine-induced effects and intrinsic drug effects. The iodine-induced effects include potentiation of thyroid autoimmunity and unregulated hormone synthesis (Jod-Basedow effect).[40] The intrinsic effects of amiodarone on the thyroid include blockade of thyroid hormone entry into the cells, decreased receptor binding of T3, and inhibition of deiodinase.[40] The most common effect of amiodarone on the fetus is hypothyroidism, although low birth weight, bradycardia, and prolongation of the QT interval can also occur.[41]

Bartalena and colleagues[42] examined the fetal effects of the administration of amiodarone to the mother. In their study, 64 neonates were exposed to amiodarone in utero. Transient hypothyroidism occurred in 17% of patients (11 out of 64); goiter developed in 3% (2 out of 64). Mental retardation and impaired speech were also noted in this patient population. These symptoms occurred in those with and without hypothyroidism. Consequently, if an alternative agent is available and appropriate, the use of amiodarone should be avoided.[41] Lidocaine and procainamide are generally considered safer than amiodarone and are the preferred pharmacologic agent for the treatment of ventricular dysrhythmias during pregnancy.[43] If amiodarone is

Table 3 Commonly used antihypertensives in pregnancy		
Class	**Name**	**Pregnancy Category**
α_2-Agonists	Clonidine	C
	Methyldopa	B
α-Antagonists	Doxazosin	C
	Phentolamine	C
	Prazosin	C
	Terazosin	C
β-Blockers	Metoprolol	C
	Nadolol	C
	Penbutolol	C
	Propranolol	C
	Carvedilol	C
Combined α- and β-blockers	Labetalol	C
	Amlodipine	C
Calcium channel blockers	Diltiazem	C
	Nicardipine	C
	Verapamil	C
	Hydrochlorothiazide	B
Miscellaneous	Hydralazine	C

administered to treat maternal dysrhythmia, surveillance for the development of a goiter through serial fetal sonograms should be performed.

Other Cardiovascular Drugs

Other cardiovascular medications are listed in **Table 3** and discussed in the article on cardiovascular disasters by Sommerkamp and Gibson elsewhere in this issue. ACLS drugs are generally considered safe.

PSYCHIATRIC MEDICATIONS
Lithium

Lithium is a monovalent cation widely used in the treatment of bipolar disorder. Several studies have associated lithium with the development of Ebstein anomaly, a congenital heart defect. Ebstein anomaly is characterized by an atrialized right ventricle in which the tricuspid valve is displaced into the right ventricle, dividing the chamber into upper (inlet) and lower (functional) portions. This displacement results in right ventricular dilation, heart failure, and arrhythmias.[44] Many of the studies establishing the association between lithium and Ebstein anomaly relied on retrospective data and various registries with the risk of reporting bias.[45] Subsequent studies have not demonstrated nearly as strong an association as once thought.[46] A recent meta-analysis failed to associate any clear association between lithium and Ebstein anomaly, although the investigators acknowledged that the exact degree of association is difficult to fully elucidate because of the rarity of this condition.[46]

DRUGS THAT ARE LIKELY NOT TERATOGENS
Anticoagulants: Unfractionated Heparin Versus Low-Molecular-Weight Heparin

The low-molecular-weight heparins, enoxaparin, dalteparin, and tinzaparin, each have an FDA pregnancy classification of B, whereas unfractionated heparin has a pregnancy classification of C. However, neither unfractionated heparin nor the low-molecular-weight heparins cross the placental barrier to any appreciable amount.[47] Consequently, either can be used in pregnancy and are preferred over vitamin K antagonists.[48,49] A recent position statement by the American College of Obstetricians and Gynecologists cites both unfractionated heparin and low-molecular-weight heparins as safe in pregnancy.[49] Although anticoagulation itself may pose risks to the mother (eg, hemorrhage, heparin-induced thrombocytopenia, osteoporosis), there is no direct teratogenic effect from either unfractionated heparin or the low-molecular-weight heparins.

ANTIMICROBIALS
Aminoglycosides

The aminoglycosides, amikacin and gentamycin, have incomplete placental transfer, meaning cord concentration is lower than that observed in maternal plasma.[50] The aminoglycosides function by binding to the bacterial 30 s ribosomal subunit and, thus, prevent bacterial protein synthesis.[51] Despite some early reports demonstrating an increased risk of fetal malformation, subsequent studies have failed to replicate the results. Animal data have revealed some dose-dependent risk of damage to the vestibular system as well as nephrotoxicity.[51] However, the doses required to produce fetal harm in animal models greatly exceeded recommended human doses.[51]

Fluoroquinolones

Quinolone and fluoroquinolone class antibiotics have become widely used to treat various infections. The fluoroquinolones inhibit bacterial topoisomerase II and, thus, block bacterial DNA replication.[51] At therapeutic doses, most fluoroquinolones are not associated with teratogenic potential. Some animal studies involving supratherapeutic doses (eg, rats receiving 810 mg/kg of levofloxacin) documented some skeletal deformities. In humans, fluoroquinolones are likely safe and are the antibiotic of choice for the treatment of certain infections during pregnancy. Several commonly used antibiotics that are safe for use during pregnancy are listed in **Table 4**.

ANTIEPILEPTICS
Benzodiazepines

Benzodiazepines are commonly prescribed for the management of anxiety and seizure disorder. Most benzodiazepines are considered category D by the FDA. Use during labor is associated with the potential for floppy infant syndrome with associated respiratory and central nervous system depression.[52] Long-term use in the third trimester is associated with the potential for fetal addiction and subsequent neonatal withdrawal.[52] Neonatal withdrawal is characterized by hypertonia, hyperreflexia, inconsolability, tremor, difficulty suckling, and abnormal sleep patterns.[53]

Several older studies examined the use of diazepam during the first trimester and found a possible association between its use and the development of cleft lip/palate in neonates.[54,55] However, larger prospective studies subsequently failed to find any association between benzodiazepines and the development of oral clefts.[53] Thus, despite the categorization of D, many of these medications are probably safe for the fetus following short-term parental administration in the ED, particularly for treatment of conditions, such as seizures or ethanol or benzodiazepine withdrawal, assuming labor is not imminent. However, if delivery is impending and the reason for administration of benzodiazepines is not life threatening (eg, status epilepticus) or if an alternative exists, then it seems reasonable to delay the administration of benzodiazepines until after delivery to reduce the likelihood of respiratory depression.

ANALGESICS
NSAIDs

Nonsteroidal antiinflammatory drugs (NSAIDs) have widespread use for their analgesic and antiinflammatory properties. These drugs are widely used in pregnancy; in one study, they were used by 23% of pregnant women.[56] Limited data suggest a small

Table 4
Acceptable antibiotics during pregnancy, by condition[a]

Condition	Antibiotics
Bacterial vaginosis	Metronidazole
Cellulitis	First- or second-generation oral cephalosporin
Chorioamnionitis	Ampicillin and gentamycin
Meningitis	Ceftriaxone and vancomycin
Pneumonia (CAP)	β-Lactam and macrolide
Skin/soft tissue	First- or second-generation oral cephalosporin
Urinary tract infection	First- or second-generation oral cephalosporin or metronidazole
Outpatient Inpatient	Ceftriaxone

Abbreviation: CAP, community-acquired pneumonia.
[a] The exact choice of antibiotics should be tailored to local sensitivity patterns.

increased risk of neural tube defects among regular users of NSAIDs compared with those who do not use these medications. The specific type of neural tube defect varies depending on which NSAID is used, and this effect was not noted in other studies.[57] Furthermore, although data are conflicting, there may be a very small increased risk of spontaneous abortion as well as cardiac malformations when NSAIDs are used early in pregnancy. However, this association is weak, and there is insufficient evidence to definitively point to a causal relationship between NSAIDs and an increased risk of either cardiac defects or miscarriage.[58] In general, many obstetricians counsel patients to avoid NSAIDs before 12 weeks of gestation because of this unclear risk. It should be noted, however, that their use in the last 6 to 8 weeks of pregnancy is contraindicated because of the association with premature closure of the ductus arteriosis,[59] which can be problematic in infants born with a ductal-dependent lesion. Consequently, it is common practice that pregnant women should not take NSAIDs before 12 and after 32 weeks of gestation.

OPIATES

Numerous studies have examined the effect of chronic opiate use throughout pregnancy. Although these drugs are not specifically teratogenic, most studies have found an increased prevalence of preterm birth and a reduction in birth weight and head circumference.[60] However, most studies did not adequately correct for confounding variables, including social situations and smoking.[61]

Long-term use of opiates can lead to neonatal abstinence syndrome, which is characterized by central nervous system abnormalities (eg, irritability, tremor, hypertonicity), vomiting, diarrhea, and tachypnea.[62] This syndrome, which can be life threatening to the newborn, is frequently managed with opiate therapy. Historically, paregoric was administered but it is no longer recommended. Oral morphine therapy is the mainstay for the treatment of neonatal opiate withdrawal[63]; but, more recently, methadone or the partial agonist buprenorphine has been used. Studies comparing methadone with buprenorphine have demonstrated that methadone is associated with somewhat longer lengths of stay and possibly a more prolonged duration of neonatal abstinence syndrome compared with buprenorphine.[64–66] Methadone must be administered cautiously and only by those with significant experience with its use. Because the maximal amount of respiratory depression may not be apparent until it manifests in a delayed fashion, there is a risk of death with rapid upward titration of the dose. Furthermore, methadone is associated with a prolongation of the QT interval, which may become problematic if patients are also taking other medications that result in blockade of the potassium efflux channels, thereby creating a potential risk of dysrhythmias caused by significant QT prolongation.

In the short term, opiate therapy is appropriate for the treatment of acute pain in pregnant women. If opiates are given shortly before birth, however, there is a risk of respiratory depression in the newborn.

COMPLICATIONS OF OBSTETRIC MANAGEMENT
Preeclampsia/Eclampsia

Preeclampsia is a multisystem disorder of the second and third trimesters of pregnancy, characterized by proteinuria and hypertension. Without treatment, preeclampsia can progress to eclampsia, the hallmark feature of which is the development of neurologic events, including seizures.[67] Pregnancy-induced hypertension, which is part of the preeclampsia and eclampsia spectrum,[68] is one of the leading causes of maternal death following live births in the United States.[69]

The optimal management of severe preeclampsia or eclampsia involves the administration of large doses of magnesium. One such dosing regimen calls for 4 g of magnesium sulfate administered intravenously over 10 to 15 minutes, followed by an infusion of 1 to 2 g/h for 24 to 48 hours.[67,70,71] The exact mechanism of action of magnesium in the management of preeclampsia or eclampsia is not definitively understood; but it is known that magnesium acts as a calcium channel antagonist, which induces cerebral vasodilatation.[67,72] Additional mechanisms of vasodilatation involve a decrease of endothelin-1 and an increase in the cyclic guanosine monophosphate concentration.

In general, high doses of magnesium are fairly well tolerated, with flushing being the most common adverse event.[71] Other commonly encountered signs of mild toxicity, which usually occur with maternal plasma magnesium concentrations between 3.8 and 5.0 mmol/L, include headaches, nystagmus, hypothermia, blurred vision, nausea, and urinary retention.[73,74] Other toxic effects can also occur and directly correlate with the plasma magnesium concentration.[73] Magnesium toxicity can have adverse effects on both the mother and the fetus. One of the first manifestations of significant maternal toxicity involves the loss of patellar reflexes, which occurs with plasma magnesium concentrations between 3.5 and 5 mmol/L.[73] Respiratory paralysis occurs at concentrations between 5.0 and 6.5 mmol/L. Cardiac conduction disturbances can occur at concentrations greater than 7.5 mmol/L, with cardiac arrest occurring at concentrations greater than 12.5 mmol/L.[73]

Treatment is largely supportive, involving airway protection as needed and fluid resuscitation. Direct-acting vasopressors can be used to treat hypotension. In addition to discontinuing the magnesium infusion, intravenous calcium can be administered to treat clinical manifestations of severe toxicity. Although either calcium gluconate or calcium chloride can be effective, calcium chloride should be administered only centrally, with very rare exceptions. One approach is the intravenous administration of 2 to 4 g of calcium gluconate over several hours.

Medical Abortions

Emergency physicians are not likely to prescribe medications for medical abortions, but they should be aware that the combination of mifepristone/misoprostol can result in a life-threatening infection. Several deaths have been reported after the combination of 200 mg of oral mifepristone and 800 mg of vaginal misoprostol.[75,76] Following the administration of these two agents to induce medical abortions, women developed a rapidly progressive septic shock, which was ultimately discovered to be caused by the gram-positive anaerobic bacillus *Clostridium sordellii*. Common characteristics in these patients included refractory hypotension, multiple effusions, and lack of fever.[75] This syndrome emerges several days after administration and occurs in greater frequency with this medicinal combination than with other preparations. If this syndrome is suspected, treatment should include the administration of broad-spectrum antibiotics, including clindamycin, and aggressive supportive care, including fluid resuscitation and vasopressors, as indicated.

SUMMARY

The emergency physician frequently encounters women who seek care because of pregnancy- and nonpregnancy-related complaints. Many medications are safe for use during pregnancy, including several that are listed as potential teratogens based on the FDA's pregnancy classification; but it is important that the emergency physician know and recognize which drugs can be given in pregnancy and which drugs are absolutely contraindicated. Expert resources should be identified and used because the FDA's classification of drugs based on pregnancy risk does not represent the most up-to-date or accurate assessment of a drug's safety.

REFERENCES

1. Ventura SJ, Abma JC, Mosher WD, et al. Estimated pregnancy rates for the United States, 1990-2005: an update. Natl Vital Stat Rep 2009;58(4):1–14.
2. Ramoska EA, Sacchetti AD, Neep M, et al. Reliability of patient history in determining the possibility of pregnancy. Ann Emerg Med 1989;18:48–50.
3. Myren M, Mose T, Mathiesen L, et al. The human placenta: an alternative for studying foetal exposure. Toxicol In Vitro 2007;21:1332–40.
4. Franks ME, Macpherson GR, Fig WD. Thalidomide. Lancet 2004;363:1802–11.
5. Lancaster PA. Causes of birth defects: lessons from history. Congenit Anom (Kyoto) 2011;51:2–5.
6. Koren G, Pastuszak A, Ito S. Drugs in pregnancy. N Engl J Med 1998;338:1128–37.
7. Daw JR, Mintzes B, Law MR, et al. Prescription drug use in pregnancy: a retrospective, population-based study in British Columbia Canada (2001-6). Clin Ther 2012;45:239–49.
8. Andrade SE, Gurwirtz JH, Davis RL, et al. Prescription drug use in pregnancy. Am J Obstet Gynecol 2004;191:398–407.
9. Walfisch A, Koren G. The "warfarin window" in pregnancy: the importance of half-life. J Obstet Gynaecol Can 2010;32:988–9.
10. Hou JW. Fetal warfarin syndrome. Chang Gung Med J 2004;27:691–5.
11. Wainwright H, Beighton P. Warfarin embryopathy: fetal manifestations. Virchows Arch 2010;457:735–9.
12. Mehndiratta S, Suneja A, Gupta B, et al. Fetotoxicity of warfarin anticoagulation. Arch Gynecol Obstet 2010;282:335–7.
13. Yerby MS. Quality of life, epilepsy advances, and the evolving role of anticonvulsants in women with epilepsy. Neurology 2000;55(5 Suppl 1):S21–31 [discussion: S54–8].
14. Battino D, Tomson T. Management of epilepsy during pregnancy. Drugs 2007;67: 2727–46.
15. Pennell PB. Antiepileptic drug pharmacokinetics during pregnancy and lactation. Neurology 2003;61(Suppl 2):S35–42.
16. Longo B, Forinash AB, Murphy JA. Levetiracetam use in pregnancy. Ann Pharmacother 2009;43:1692–5.
17. Jentink J, Dolk H, Loane MA, et al. Intrauterine exposure to carbamazepine and specific congenital malformations: systemic review and case-control study. BMJ 2010;341:c6581.
18. Speidel BD, Meadow SR. Maternal epilepsy and abnormalities of the fetus and newborn. Lancet 1972;2:839–43.
19. Holmes LB. Teratogen-induced limb defects. Am J Med Genet 2002;112:297–303.
20. Eadie MJ. Antiepileptic drugs as human teratogens. Expert Opin Drug Saf 2008; 7:195–209.
21. Wyszynski DF, Nambisan M, Surve T, et al. Increased rate of major malformations in offspring exposed to valproate during pregnancy. Neurology 2005;64:961–5.
22. Kozma C. Valproic acid embryopathy: report of two siblings with further expansion of the phenotypic abnormalities and a review of the literature. Am J Med Genet 2001;98:168–75.

23. Robert E, Guibaud P. Maternal valproic acid and congenital neural tube defects. Lancet 1982;2:937.
24. Hyuon S, Obican SG, Scialli AR. Teratogen update: methotrexate. Birth Defects Res A Clin Mol Teratol 2012;94:187–207.
25. Poogi SH, Ghidini A. Importance of timing of gestational exposure to methotrexate for its teratogenic effects when used in setting of misdiagnosis of ectopic pregnancy. Fertil Steril 2011;96:669–71.
26. Nurmohamed L, Moretti ME, Schechter T. Outcome following high-dose methotrexate in pregnancies misdiagnosed as ectopic. Am J Obstet Gynecol 2011; 205:533.e1–3.
27. Kutscher AH, Zagarelli EV, Tovell HM, et al. Discoloration of teeth induced by tetracycline administered ante partum. JAMA 1963;184:586–7.
28. Harcourt JK, Johnson NW, Storey E. In vivo incorporation of tetracycline in the teeth of man. Arch Oral Biol 1962;7:421–7.
29. Czeizel AE, Rocckenbauer M. Teratogenic study of doxycycline. Obstet Gynecol 1997;89:524–8.
30. Cooper WO, Hernandez-Diaz S, Arbogast PG, et al. Antibiotics potentially used in response to bioterrorism and the risk of major congenital malformations. Paediatr Perinat Epidemiol 2009;23:18–28.
31. Kazy E, Puho EH, Czeizel AE. Effect of doxycycline treatment during pregnancy for birth outcomes. Reprod Toxicol 2007;24:279–80.
32. Tetracycline. Micromedex. Available at: www.thomsonhc.com/micromedex2/librarian/ND_T/evidencexpert/ND_PR/evidencexpert/CS/DD2C0F/ND_AppProduct/evidencexpert/DUPLICATIONSHIELDSYNC/BF551D/ND_PG/evidencexpert/ND_B/evidencexpert/ND_P/evidencexpert/PFActionId/evidencexpert.DisplayDrugdexDocument?docId=0557&;contentSetId=31&title=Tetracycline&servicesTitle=Tetracycline&topicId=cautionsSection&subtopicId=teratogenicityEffectsInPregnancyBreastfeedingSection. Accessed April 18, 2012.
33. Maron BA, Rocco TP. Chapter 28. Pharmacotherapy of congestive heart failure. In: Chabner BA, Brunton LL, Knollman BC, editors. Goodman & Gilman's the pharmacological basis of therapeutics. 12th edition. New York: McGraw-Hill Medical; 2011. Available at: http://www.accesspharmacy.com/content.aspx?aID=16668047. Accessed September 28, 2012.
34. Piper JM, Ray WA, Rosa FW. Pregnancy outcome following exposure to angiotensin-converting enzyme inhibitors. Obstet Gynecol 1992;80(3 Pt 1):429–32.
35. Tabacova S, Little R, Tsong Y, et al. Adverse pregnancy outcomes associated with maternal enalapril antihypertensive treatment. Pharmacoepidemiol Drug Saf 2003;12:633–46.
36. Pyrde PG, Sedman AB, Nugent CE, et al. Angiotensin-converting enzyme inhibitor fetopathy. J Am Soc Nephrol 1993;3:1575–82.
37. Schaefer C. Angiotensin II receptor antagonists: further evidence of fetotoxicity but not teratogenicity. Birth Defects Res A Clin Mol Teratol 2003;67:591–4.
38. Cooper WO, Hernandez-Diaz S, Arbogast PG, et al. Major congenital malformations after first-trimester exposure to ACE inhibitors. N Engl J Med 2006;354: 2443–51.
39. Singh BN. Current antiarrhythmic drugs: an overview of mechanisms of action and potential clinical utility. J Cardiovasc Electrophysiol 1999;10:283–301.
40. Padmanabhan H. Amiodarone and thyroid dysfunction. South Med J 2010;103: 922–30.
41. Joglar JA, Page RL. Antiarrhythmic drugs in pregnancy. Curr Opin Cardiol 2011; 16:40–5.

42. Bartalena L, Bogazzi F, Braverman LE, et al. Effects of amiodarone administration during pregnancy on neonatal thyroid function and subsequent neurodevelopment. J Endocrinol Invest 2001;24:116–30.
43. Gowda RM, Khan IA, Mehta NJ, et al. Cardiac arrhythmias in pregnancy: clinical and therapeutic considerations. Int J Cardiol 2003;88:129–33.
44. Attenhofer Jost CH, Connolly HM, Dearnari JA, et al. Ebstein's anomaly. Circulation 2007;115:277–85.
45. Matok I, Pupco A, Koren G, et al. Drug exposure in pregnancy and heart disease. J Cardiovasc Pharmacol 2011;58:20–4.
46. McNight RF, Adida M, Budge K, et al. Lithium toxicity profile: a systemic review and meta-analysis. Lancet 2012;379:721–8.
47. Ramin SM, Ramin KD, Gilstrap LC. Anticoagulants and thrombolytics during pregnancy. Semin Perinatol 1997;21:149–53.
48. Bates SM, Greer IA, Pabinger I. Venous thromboembolism, thrombophilia, antithrombotic therapy, and pregnancy: American College of Chest Physicians evidence-based clinical practice guidelines, 8th ed. Chest 2008;136: 844S–86S.
49. James A, Committee on Practice Bulletins – Obstetrics. Practice bulletin No. 123: thromboembolism in pregnancy. Obstet Gynecol 2011;118:718–29.
50. Pacifici GM. Placental transfer of antibiotics administered to the mother: a review. Int J Clin Pharmacol Ther 2006;44:57–63.
51. Nahum GG, Uhl K, Kennedy DL. Antibiotic use in pregnancy and lactation: what is and is not known about teratogenic and toxic risks. Obstet Gynecol 2006;107: 1120–38.
52. McElhatton PR. The effects of benzodiazepine use during pregnancy and lactation. Reprod Toxicol 1995;8:461–75.
53. Iqbal MM, Sobhan T, Ryals T. Effects of commonly used benzodiazepines on the fetus, the neonate, and the nursing infant. Psychiatr Serv 2002;53:39–49.
54. Aaroskg D. Letter: association between maternal intake of diazepam and oral clefts. Lancet 1975;2:921.
55. Saxen I, Saxen L. Letter: association between maternal intake of diazepam and oral clefts. Lancet 1975;13:498.
56. Werler MM, Mitchell AA, Hernandez-Diaz S, et al. Use of over-the-counter medications during pregnancy. Am J Obstet Gynecol 2005;193:771–7.
57. Hernandez RK, Werler MM, Romitti P, et al. Nonsteroidal anti-inflammatory drug use among women and the risk of birth defects. Am J Obstet Gynecol 2012; 206:228.e1–8.
58. Chambers CD, Tutuncu ZN, Johnson D, et al. Human pregnancy safety for agents used to treat rheumatoid arthritis: adequacy of available information and strategies for developing post-marketing data. Arthritis Res Ther 2006;8:215.
59. Risser A, Donovan D, Heintzman J, et al. NSAID prescribing precautions. Am Fam Physician 2009;80:1371–8.
60. Minnes S, Lang A, Singer L. Prenatal tobacco, marijuana, stimulant, and opiate exposure: outcomes and practice implications. Addict Sci Clin Pract 2011;6: 57–70.
61. Schempf AH. Illicit drug use and neonatal outcomes: a critical review. Obstet Gynecol Surv 2007;62:749–57.
62. Johnson K, Cerada C, Greenough A. Treatment of neonatal abstinence syndrome. Arch Dis Child Fetal Neonatal Ed 2003;88:F2–5.
63. Bio LL, Siu A, Poon CY. Update on the pharmacologic management of neonatal abstinence syndrome. J Perinatol 2001;31:692–701.

64. Jones HE, Johnson RE, Jasinski DR, et al. Buprenorphine versus methadone in the treatment of pregnant opioid-dependent patients: effects on the neonatal abstinence syndrome. Drug Alcohol Depend 2005;79:1–10.

65. Jones HE, Kaltenbach K, Heil SH, et al. Neonatal abstinence syndrome after methadone or buprenorphine exposure. N Engl J Med 2010;363:2320–31.

66. Lacroix I, Berrebi A, Garipuy D, et al. Buprenorphine versus methadone in pregnant opioid-dependent women: a prospective multicenter study. Eur J Clin Pharmacol 2011;67:1053–9.

67. McCoy S, Baldwin K. Pharmacotherapeutic options for the treatment of preeclampsia. Am J Health Syst Pharm 2009;66:337–44.

68. Leeman L, Fontaine P. Hypertensive disorders of pregnancy. Am Fam Physician 2008;78:93–100.

69. Chang J, Elam-Evans LD, Berg CJ, et al. Pregnancy-related mortality surveillance – United States, 1991-1999. MMWR Surveill Summ 2003;52:1–8.

70. Lowe SA, Brown MA, Dekker GA, et al. Guidelines for the management of hypertensive disorders of pregnancy 2008. Aust N Z J Obstet Gynaecol 2009;49: 242–6.

71. Duley L, Gulmezoglu AM, Henderson-Smart DJ, et al. Magnesium sulfate and other anticonvulsants for women with pre-eclampsia. Cochrane Database Syst Rev 2010;(11):CD000025.

72. James MF. Magnesium in obstetrics. Best Pract Res Clin Obstet Gynaecol 2010; 24:327–37.

73. Lu JF, Nightingale CH. Magnesium sulfate in eclampsia and pre-eclampsia. Clin Pharm 2000;38:305–14.

74. Sibai BM. Magnesium sulfate prophylaxis in preeclampsia: evidence from randomized trials. Clin Obstet Gynecol 2005;48:478–88.

75. Fischer M, Bhatnagar J, Guarner J, et al. Fatal toxic shock syndrome associated with Clostridium sordellii after medical abortion. N Engl J Med 2005;353:2352–60.

76. Centers for Disease Control and Prevention (CDC). Clostridium sordellii toxic shock syndrome after medical abortion with mifepristone and intravaginal misoprostol—United States and Canada—2001–2005. MMWR Morb Mortal Wkly Rep 2005;54:724.

Emergency Evaluation and Management of Vaginal Bleeding in the Nonpregnant Patient

Angela R. Cirilli, MD, RDMS*, Stephen J. Cipot, DO

KEYWORDS

- Vaginal bleeding • Fibroids • Endometriosis • Abnormal uterine bleeding
- Dysfunctional uterine bleeding • Menorrhagia • Progesterone

KEY POINTS

- The chief complaint of vaginal bleeding includes a broad differential, including pregnancy and pregnancy-related problems, underlying structural uterine pathology, and abnormal uterine bleeding without a known cause.
- Fibroids are common in many women with abnormal bleeding and can be diagnosed adequately with ultrasound in the emergency department.
- Endometriosis is a difficult diagnosis to make, but physicians need to maintain a high degree of suspicion for it in patients presenting with pain and bleeding.
- *Dysfunctional uterine bleeding* is a catch-all term with various interpretations. It should be changed to *abnormal uterine bleeding*, referring to both anovulatory and ovulatory bleeding disturbances.
- Several medical options are available for the treatment of abnormal uterine bleeding. Hysterectomy is a last resort for those who have no wish for further fertility and for whom medical treatment was not successful.

INTRODUCTION

Managing vaginal bleeding in the nonpregnant patient can be difficult for many emergency physicians because of the wide array of potential causes and the unfamiliar nature of management options. Sources of bleeding range from fibroids to endometriosis, and abnormal uterine bleeding can have anovulatory and ovulatory hormonal causes (**Box 1**). Pregnancy must always be ruled out. It is the job of the emergency physician to be aware of the rare life-threatening complications associated with these diagnoses that require emergent surgery and to rule out life-threatening anemia when

The authors received no financial support or gifts related to the preparation of this article.
Department of Emergency Medicine, Northshore University Hospital, 300 Community Drive, Manhasset, NY 11030, USA
* Corresponding author.
E-mail address: angcirilli@gmail.com

Box 1
Differential diagnosis for abnormal uterine bleeding

Pregnancy/pregnancy-related bleeding

Structural problems

  Atrioventricular malformation

  Polyps

  Fibroids

  Endometriosis

  Hyperplasia

Coagulopathies (ie, von Willebrand disease)

Polycystic ovarian syndrome

Intrauterine or oral contraceptives

Medications (antiepileptics, typical and atypical antipsychotics)

Endometritis (gonorrhea, chlamydial infection)

---

bleeding is severe. Obstetric consultation can be obtained, with imaging as an outpatient, unless life-threatening complications are suspected.

FIBROIDS (UTERINE MYOMAS)
Epidemiology and Pathophysiology

Fibroids are benign, often asymptomatic, tumors that occur within the uterus. Fibroids are the most common pelvic tumor in the gynecologic patient population. Prevalence studies estimate that from 20% to nearly half of American women in their reproductive years have uterine fibroids, and the majority are asymptomatic.[1] The occurrence appears to increase with age. It is also higher in African Americans than in Caucasians, with a cumulative occurrence of 80% in African Americans and 70% in whites and by age 50 years.[1] Most fibroids are asymptomatic; therefore, the emergency physician needs to determine whether the cause of vaginal bleeding or lower abdominal pain is a symptomatic fibroid or a more serious condition.

Etiology

The exact cause of fibroids is unknown. Fibroid growth is largely dependent on steroid hormones and genetic factors. The hormones that have been implicated in fibroid physiology are estrogen, progestin, and gonadotropin-releasing hormone agonists (GnRH-a).[2] Historically, decreased estrogen concentration was believed to be the independent cause of the postmenopausal decrease in fibroid growth.[3] However, it is now known that an increased level of GnRH-a during menopause suppresses release of estrogen and progestin from ovarian follicles.[4] Therefore, the growth of fibroids depends on progestin, estrogen, and GnRH-a balance. This physiology plays an important role in tailoring pharmacologic therapies to suppress fibroid growth.

Symptoms, Diagnosis, and Management

The Federation International d'Obstetrique et Gynecologie (FIGO) classification system is widely accepted and defines the position of fibroids within the uterine wall.[5] Fibroids are classified as SM (at least 1 submucosal lesion) or O (all intramural or subserosal layer). Most clinically relevant fibroids are submucosal.

The symptoms of fibroids vary from common complaints of abnormal uterine bleeding to rare presentations related to excessive growth and mass effect on adjacent organs (**Table 1**).[6] Fibroids can present with a combination of symptoms, making the diagnosis challenging. In a young female with acute pain and vaginal bleeding, it becomes more important to eliminate an ectopic pregnancy as a cause than to diagnose a fibroid, except in rare circumstances.

Physical Examination

The physical examination of a patient presenting with a fibroid will vary based on her symptoms and the size of the tumor. Large fibroids can sometimes be palpated during the abdominal and rectal examinations. The patient may have lower abdominal tenderness if the peritoneal cavity has been irritated by free pelvic fluid or if pain is being referred from the uterus.[7] A bimanual examination may reveal clotted dark blood. Although physical examinations are necessary, they usually do not contribute to the diagnosis of a uterine fibroid.

Diagnostic Testing

The best screening test for most pelvic complaints is ultrasonography. Although the diagnosis of a fibroid is emergent in only a few circumstances, an ultrasound examination should be performed in cases of severe pain and bleeding to rule out serious diagnosis such as hemorrhagic cysts, ovarian torsion, ectopic pregnancy, and the rare case of a degenerating or torqued fibroid. Most sonographically diagnosed fibroids are found incidentally while looking for other emergent pelvic diagnoses.

In sonographic terms a fibroid is described as a hypoechoic mass originating from the uterine wall with well-defined borders. Fibroids may have mixed echogenicity with hyperechoic calcifications causing poster shadowing and some hypoechoic areas.[8] Images should be correlated with the location of the fibroid. Using color flow Doppler can help decipher whether the blood supply to the fibroid has been disrupted. A degenerating fibroid will appear more cystic. In rare circumstances, magnetic resonance imaging (MRI) is performed if bedside ultrasonography is nondiagnostic, and is almost never needed emergently. When further imaging is necessary, MRI is preferred over computed tomography (CT) to avoid unnecessary radiation in the characteristically young population. In general, emergent imaging of fibroids is not necessary and can be done on an outpatient basis, unless the patient has severe pain or peritoneal signs suggesting rare but serious complications, or a diagnosis unrelated to fibroids.

A urine or serum pregnancy test is mandatory to rule out ectopic pregnancy as the cause of the patient's pain. Other laboratory tests should be evaluated and correlated with the diagnosis of fibroids as deemed necessary by the emergency physician.

Table 1	
Symptoms of uterine fibroids	
Symptom	**Cause**
Abnormal uterine bleeding	Disruption of the submucosal blood supply surrounding the fibroid, often during menstruation
Infertility and miscarriage	Failure of implantation or disruption of the implanted fetus
Acute pain	Degeneration or twisting of the blood supply to a fibroid, causing ischemia of the fibroid
Chronic/indolent pain	A growing fibroid that extends into local layers and stretches pain fibers
Constipation/urinary retention	A local mass effect on adjacent bowel, bladder, or urethra

Hemoglobin and hematocrit may be useful in a patient with heavy or prolonged bleeding but are not absolutely necessary if severe anemia is not suspected. A total white blood cell count, although nonspecific, may point toward another diagnosis such as pelvic inflammatory disease or a tubo-ovarian abscess, but is likely to be noncontributory to the diagnosis of fibroids. In the majority of cases, laboratory evaluation is nonspecific and will be noncontributory in diagnosing fibroids, and can be limited to a urine pregnancy test.

Management

The management of uncomplicated uterine fibroids depends on the severity and duration of the patient's symptoms, and is primarily expectant. Management can be divided into medical and procedural options (**Table 2**). It is generally preferred to manage patients with fibroids expectantly and provide the least invasive treatment options first. From a public health perspective, women who choose to be treated more aggressively often incur higher health care and social costs than those who seek medical treatment alone.[9]

In the emergency department (ED), management should focus on differentiating patients with acute emergent complications associated with fibroids from those with long-standing uncomplicated or even asymptomatic fibroids. Although acute complications from fibroids are very rare, they do include conditions such as a torsed

Table 2 Fibroid management	
Medical Management	
Nonsteroidal anti-inflammatory drugs (NSAIDs)	Symptomatic control is the first and best option for controlling pain and bleeding attributed to fibroids. Patients can have a 30% reduction in blood loss. There is less cost and morbidity associated with NSAID therapy than with procedural management.[53]
Gonadotropin-releasing hormone agonists (leuprolide)	Decreases estrogen and progestin, causing a perimenopause state. The adverse effect of concern is osteopenia. Add-back therapy with estrogen helps mitigate this effect. Short-term therapy can cause a 55% reduction in the size of fibroids[54]
Antiprogestins (mifepristone)	A reduction in the size and even elimination of uterine fibroids[55]
Procedural Management	
Myomectomy	Myomectomy can be done via laparoscopy or laparotomy. Indications for myomectomy are largely being called into question as more studies demonstrate that patient complaints may not correlate with the fibroid demonstrated by examination or ultrasonography[6]
Uterine artery embolization	An alternative to women requesting the definitive therapy for hysterectomy. A Cochrane review concluded that it provides similar results as hysterectomy and sometimes myomectomy. Recovery time is reduced; however, some women experience more pain[56]
Hysterectomy	Indications for total abdominal hysterectomy are symptoms severe enough to be socially debilitating. Severe complications occur in 3% of patients[57]

pedunculated fibroid, acute vaginal or intraperitoneal hemorrhage, urinary retention from obstruction (usually seen when they increase in size during pregnancy), deep vein thrombosis leading to pulmonary embolism from vascular compression, and mesenteric thrombosis from mechanical compression resulting in intestinal necrosis.[10]

Patients with acute fibroid torsion or intraperitoneal hemorrhage usually present with an acute abdomen and may require emergent exploratory laparotomy. Severe anemia from vaginal or intraperitoneal hemorrhage secondary to fibroids is also very rare, but may require emergent transfusion. The most common presentation of abnormal bleeding secondary to fibroids is chronic menorrhagia, causing iron-deficiency anemia.[11] Patients with long-standing uterine fibroids should be referred to a gynecologist on an outpatient basis or started on hormonal agents if proper consultation can be arranged within the ED. The use of nonsteroidal anti-inflammatory drugs (NSAIDs) can be initiated by the emergency physician safely in patients at low risk for complications such as gastric bleeding.

Summary

Uterine fibroids are common tumors of the uterus that can cause pelvic pain, bleeding, and infertility. Growth depends on several physiologic hormones that are active during a woman's reproductive life span. Despite their common nature, most fibroids are asymptomatic; therefore, identification of a uterine fibroid on ultrasonography in a woman with associated symptoms does not necessarily mean that the fibroid is the cause of her presentation to the ED. The ED physician should be diligent in providing pain relief and eliminating the possibility of other serious or life-threatening complications, especially related to pregnancy The ED physician should educate patients regarding expectant management with regard to fibroid treatment. The risks of surgical intervention for a benign fibroid far outweigh the benefits. Emergency physicians must be knowledgable about uterine fibroids, as they are highly prevalent and are a potential cause of pelvic or abdominal pain, bleeding, and miscarriages.

ENDOMETRIOSIS

Endometriosis is a diagnosis that must be considered by emergency physicians when presented with a patient who complains of pelvic pain, dysmenorrhea, dyspareunia, or abnormal uterine bleeding. Although life-threatening complications such as vital-organ implants or bowel perforation are very rare, suspicion should be high in patients with a history of disease and severe symptoms or examination findings. In most cases, ED management consists of pain control and appropriate outpatient consultation.

Epidemiology and Pathophysiology

Endometriosis is defined as the presence of productive endometrial tissue and glands outside the uterine cavity. It is a chronic disease that mimics many features of malignancy. Endometrial implants can be found anywhere throughout the pelvic cavity, on the ovaries, on the uterine ligament, and even at distant sites, including the lung and pleural cavities.[12] The prevalence of endometriosis in the general population is difficult to estimate because it is a diagnosis typically made in the operating room. It is estimated that between 3% and 10% of women of reproductive age have endometriosis.[13] In patients with chronic pelvic pain who are undergoing laparoscopy, the prevalence of endometriosis can be as high as 47% to 67%. In addition, patients suffering from dysmenorrhea are 80% more likely to be diagnosed with endometriosis.[14]

Endometriosis is a disease of significant morbidity, as it causes pelvic pain, dysmenorrhea, painful intercourse, and infertility. The disease process itself can be intractable, leading to significant social, physical, and emotional burdens. There is a high rate of hospital admission for pain control and surgical procedures secondary to endometriosis. Patients with endometriosis report missing an average of 33.6 days of work annually and 19.3 days related to treatment, surgery, and recovery.[15] The rate of work absenteeism for endometriosis is higher than for headaches, arthritis, and back pain.[16]

Etiology

The cause of endometriosis is uncertain. The long-standing hypothesis is that retrograde menstruation disseminates endometrial implants to areas outside the uterus.[17] Endometrial cells attach to the pelvic cavity and grow in response to the hormones of menstruation and then self-perpetuate by releasing cytokines and growth factors. Growth of these lesions is then dependent on their blood supply, which is related to a patient's genetic predisposition and environmental factors.

In adolescents, anatomic defects that prevent or impair the outflow of menstruation, such as obstructive Müllerian anomalies, can precipitate the retrograde flow that causes endometriosis.[18] Iatrogenic dissemination of endometrial tissue can also occur during a surgical cesarean section when a surgeon inadvertently introduces tissue into a scar or the abdominal wall.[19]

Some of these implants undergo inflammatory and fibrotic changes, transforming the lesion into an endometrioma, or a "chocolate cyst." Developed endometriomas can produce scarring and adhesions within the pelvis and abdomen.[20] These lesions can vary within the same individual as much as across patients. Factors determining which lesions are clinically significant or painful include the extent of invasion, the synthesis of prostaglandins, and the vascularity of the lesions.

The majority of implants are found in the dependent portions of the pelvis, most commonly in the ovaries. The cervix, vagina, and other parts of lower genital tract are also possible areas for implants. Lymphatic involvement occurs in 30% of women. Advanced disease, whereby bowel and lungs can be affected, occurs in 10% of women.[21]

Symptoms

Endometriosis should always be on the differential diagnosis for a female patient presenting with chronic lower abdominal pain. Because the tissue implants are hormonally responsive, pain correlates with the menstrual cycle. Although most patients are asymptomatic, the classic triad of endometriosis is dysmenorrhea, infertility, and dyspareunia.[22] Dysmenorrhea is the most common symptom and precedes menstruation. Infertility can affect 30% to 50% of women.[23] Symptoms also include abnormal uterine bleeding, chronic pelvic pain, lower back pain, dyschezia, and dysuria. Several case reports have described endometriosis leading to bowel perforation.[24] Although these are rare scenarios, a patient presenting with peritoneal signs and a history of endometriosis warrants proper surgical consultation. Symptoms are summarized in **Table 3**.

One would think that the symptoms of endometriosis directly correlate with the extent of disease. However, recent studies demonstrate that correlating the extent of infiltration and symptoms is difficult. In fact, patients with relatively small endometrial implants can experience debilitating symptoms.[25]

Physical Examination

Endometriosis is rarely diagnosed in the ED because the cardinal physical examination findings and diagnostic imaging carry low sensitivities and specificities. Physical

Table 3	
Symptoms of endometriosis	
Dysmenorrhea	Most common symptom
Infertility	Affects 30%–50% of women
Dyspareunia	
Dysfunctional uterine bleeding	
Chronic pelvic pain	
Low back pain	
Dyschezia	
Dysuria	
Peritoneal signs	Seen in rare cases involving bowel perforation caused by endometriosis

examination findings include tenderness along the uterosacral ligament, a retroverted uterus, uterine pain during bimanual examination, and rectovaginal nodularity.

Diagnostic Imaging

Ultrasonography may be helpful in diagnosing ovarian endometriomas, which appear as unilocular cystic structures within the ovary and demonstrate internal echoes.[26] However, ultrasonography has a reported overall sensitivity of 11% for visualizing endometrial implants.[27] CT scans carry a sensitivity of 15% in identifying endometriosis.[28] MRI is the best noninvasive modality in diagnosing endometriosis, with an overall sensitivity of 69% and specificity of 75%.[29] The overall gold standard for diagnosis of endometriosis is under direct visualization via laparoscopy or laparotomy.

Management

The management of endometriosis is individualized and targeted to whether the patient presents with pain, infertility, or a pelvic mass. Pain is often divided into mild, moderate, and severe. Medical management is the first-line therapy for women with mild forms of endometriosis. Pelvic pain and dysmenorrhea are often caused by prostaglandin synthesis, which can be moderated with NSAIDs. Patients experiencing mild pain may report improvement within 3 days to 1 week.[30]

Hormonal therapy induces a state of amenorrhea and can be initiated with the consultation of a gynecologist, if available, in the ED. However, most of these regimens will be started by a gynecologist on an outpatient basis, as these medicines require follow-up. Oral medroxyprogesterone acetate is the most common oral contraceptive used to induce a pregnancy-like state to shrink endometrial implants. Leuprolide acetate (Lupron) is a GnRH-a that is also used to downregulate the growth of endometriomas. Patients recently started on this medication may present to the ED with the complaint of an increase in symptoms. These patients should be advised that this is an expected outcome because the pituitary gland releases hormones active in the development of endometriosis before the downregulatory effect of the medication. Leuprolide is indicated for a maximum of only 6 months before a hormonal add-back therapy is initiated, as it may precipitate osteoporosis.[30]

Outpatient surgical management is indicated for failed medical therapy or secondary infertility. Laparoscopic surgery entails visualizing and destroying or resecting these implants. Surgical resection can lessen the time to conception for infertile patients.[31] Local control of endometrial implants to preserve ovarian function and pelvic anatomy is preferred over total abdominal hysterectomy and bilateral salpingo-oophorectomy (TAH-BSO). TAH-BSO is the definitive therapy for endometriosis but is reserved for patients who no longer wish to have children or in whom the conservative approach is not successful. The management of endometriosis is summarized in **Table 4**.

Emergent surgical consultation from a gynecologist or general surgeon needs to be initiated from the ED when examination findings suggest a ruptured bowel secondary to intestinal implants or other serious complications.

Summary

Endometriosis is a chronic disease characterized by cyclical pelvic pain and infertility. The length of time between the onset of symptoms and diagnosis can be 3 to 20 years.[32] Much of this time is accounted for by improper identification of patients in need of gynecologic referral and lack of accurate, definitive testing, aside from laparoscopy, to confirm the diagnosis.

The job of the emergency physician is to identify patients with clinical descriptions that match potential endometriosis so that proper outpatient referral to a gynecologist can be made and outpatient medical therapy can be initiated when warranted. Emergency physicians should also maintain a high degree of suspicion in a patient with a history of endometriosis and severe abdominal examination findings suggestive of bowel perforation secondary to possible implants. Aside from NSAIDs, medical therapy should be initiated in consultation with a gynecologist, and can be started on an outpatient basis. A high degree of suspicion and appropriate referral will improve the morbidity rate for patients who may otherwise go undiagnosed for most of their reproductive years.

DYSFUNCTIONAL OR ABNORMAL UTERINE BLEEDING

Dysfunctional uterine bleeding is a term that has been used traditionally to describe abnormal, irregular, and heavy vaginal bleeding without a known structural or physiologic cause. There is as much confusion in the ED on how to diagnose this problem and what to do about it as there is on an international level regarding how to define it. It has been suggested by the International Federation of Obstetrics and Gynecology that the term *dysfunctional uterine bleeding* be discarded secondary to the lack of consensus surrounding what the term actually means.[33] Many physicians consider dysfunctional bleeding to be heavy, prolonged, or irregular bleeding in the nonpregnant patient, which is not related to a structural anatomic problem such as fibroids or polyps or a physiologic coagulopathy.

Table 4 Management of endometriosis	
Medical	
NSAIDs	Decrease prostaglandin synthesis
Hormonal agents	
Medroxyprogesterone acetate	Induces amenorrhea
Leuprolide acetate (Lupron)	GnRH agonist
Surgical	
Local laparoscopic resection of implants	
Total abdominal hysterectomy and bilateral salpingo-oophoerectomy	Definitive treatment, causes permanent infertility

In the United States, the term often refers to irregular nonovulatory bleeding that is not necessarily heavy but is very irregular, and may range from infrequent or missed periods to heavy intermenstrual bleeding. In most other countries, dysfunctional uterine bleeding refers to both anovulatory and ovulatory bleeding. Many agree that the term should be *abnormal uterine bleeding*, which encompasses both anovulatory and ovulatory bleeding in women of reproductive years. For the sake of discussion it is referred to here as abnormal uterine bleeding, specifically discussing prolonged and heavy premenopausal bleeding in the nonpregnant patient.

Etiology

The causes of abnormal uterine bleeding are different, depending on whether it is anovulatory or ovulatory. Anovulatory uterine bleeding is caused by a disruption of the hypothalamic-pituitary-ovarian axis. It usually occurs at the extremes of reproductive ages from unopposed estrogen and its effects on the endometrium, with lack of opposing progesterone released during ovulation.[34] The effects of unopposed estrogen on the endometrium cause the following:

- Endometrial hyperplasia
- Decreased vascular tone directly and indirectly via disturbed angiogenesis
- Inhibition of prostaglandins

The most common cause of anovulatory bleeding is polycystic ovarian disease, which is a separate entity and is not discussed here.

Ovulatory bleeding is sometimes referred to as menorrhagia (both acute and chronic) and involves heavy or prolonged bleeding in association with the menstrual cycle (usually heaviest on days 1–3).

Patient History

The most important tool to characterize, diagnose, and manage abnormal uterine bleeding is a detailed history regarding the flow disturbance. It is important to ask women whether they experience chronic heavy or prolonged bleeding at time of their cycle, intermenstrual bleeding, spotting after or before a cycle, or acute severe bleeding. In women who describe heavy blood loss (traditionally, >80 mL is considered menorrhagia), it may be useful to ask about the presence of clots, the number of pad/tampon changes, and history of anemia, as these may be better predictors of actual increases in blood loss.[35] Concurrent use of contraceptives, the presence of an intrauterine device, and a history of fibroids or endometriosis should also be elicited, as these are other causes of abnormal uterine bleeding. Recent exposure to, a history of, or risk factors for sexually transmitted diseases should also be ascertained, as chronic endometritis from gonorrhea or chlamydial infection can cause irregular intermenstrual bleeding.

The patient's medication list should be evaluated. A few drugs, such as antiepileptics (especially valproic acid), are associated with anovulatory abnormal bleeding. Commonly used typical antipsychotics (eg, haloperidol, chlorpromazine, thiothixene [Navane]) can lead to hyperandrogenism and anovulation.[36] In addition, atypical antipsychotics can contribute to anovulation by raising prolactin levels and secondary abnormal bleeding. These medications include, but are not limited to, the most common offender risperidone (Risperdal) and, less commonly, clozapine (Clozaril) and others in its class.[37]

Emergency Department Workup

There is not much consensus on the initial ED evaluation and workup for patients with abnormal uterine bleeding. Several algorithms have been established for evaluation of abnormal uterine bleeding in the outpatient setting, but little has been published regarding guidelines for ED evaluation. In general, the workup should involve a detailed history to elucidate the type of abnormal bleeding (either ovulatory or anovulatory and chronic vs acute). Appropriate evaluation for stability and resuscitation may be necessary when bleeding is severe. Imaging and consultation with a gynecologist depend on severity of the bleeding and the patient's access to follow-up.

Laboratory Tests

- Initial workup
  - Complete blood count (CBC) with platelets
  - Coagulation studies
  - Pregnancy test
  - Thyroid-stimulating hormone
  - Platelet function analysis (if the history suggests an abnormality)

Pregnancy and anemia should be ruled out. Systemic causes of bleeding such as liver failure, renal failure causing platelet dysfunction, and hypothyroidism should be considered. Testing for these should be done in the ED only if other symptoms or physical examination findings suggest the diagnosis. In younger adolescent patients with severe bleeding at the onset of menarche, von Willebrand disease should be considered. However, it is unlikely that a 20- to 30-year-old patient or a patient presenting in the perimenopausal age range would have an undiagnosed coagulopathy.

Anemia

The percentage of patients who present to the ED with abnormal vaginal bleeding and are actually anemic is unknown. A recent study that looked for an association between menorrhagia and hemoglobin levels found that bleeding longer than 7 days was the only significant predictor for a decrease in hemoglobin.[38] Another outpatient-based study evaluating current practice patterns found that up to 46% of presenting women with abnormal bleeding who reported heavy bleeding and underwent a CBC were actually anemic (hemoglobin level <7.5 mmol/L). Not all of the patients in the study were evaluated with a CBC, and the practicing physicians were able to order a CBC without objective criteria.[39]

If the clinical history and presentation suggest severe blood loss or symptoms of anemia, such as fatigue or shortness of breath, or signs of hemodynamic instability on presentation, a CBC should be obtained in the ED. For patients presenting with severe acute bleeding, transfusion may be necessary if they are unstable or symptomatic.

Management

In patients presenting with abnormal bleeding, the following stepwise pattern can be used:

1. Rule out pregnancy
2. Assess hemodynamic stability
   a. Hemodynamically stable
      i. If the patient has no signs or symptoms of anemia, recommend outpatient referral and ultrasonography to rule out structural abnormalities
      ii. If the patient has no access to health care, consider ED consultation and imaging if available
   b. Hemodynamically unstable
      i. Active resuscitation and laboratory evaluation to rule out anemia and coagulopathy

ii. Transfusion if necessary

iii. Emergent obstetric consultation

iv. Ultrasound imaging to rule out structural abnormalities such as leiomyomas

v. Admission for patients who have severe continuous bleeding while in the ED

Diagnostic Evaluation

Transvaginal ultrasonography is the diagnostic test of choice in premenopausal women with abnormal bleeding to rule out underlying structural causes such as fibroids and polyps.[40] One study reported these structural abnormalities in as many as 41% of patients presenting with abnormal uterine bleeding.[39] The procedure can be performed easily in the ED in addition to a detailed examination, including speculum and bimanual examinations, to evaluate for visible abnormalities such as trauma, cervical polyps, and lacerations.

Other tests such as MRI or hysterosonographic evaluation with saline infusion may be needed on an outpatient basis to evaluate for underlying abnormality not detected on transvaginal ultrasonography; these studies are not practical in the ED. Women with risk factors for endometrial carcinoma or hyperplasia should receive referral for outpatient evaluation, including endometrial biopsy, to rule out cancer. Perimenopausal bleeding is associated with carcinoma in 10% of women. Endometrial thickness on ultrasound imaging in premenopausal women is an inaccurate predictor for cancer. Therefore, assessment for risk factors such as obesity (weight >90 kg) and age older than 40 years should prompt referral for further workup and potential biopsy. Other risk factors for endometrial cancer include nulliparity, history of anovulatory cycles, tamoxifen use, infertility, and a family history of endometrial or colon cancer.[41]

Medical Management

In general, medical therapies for the patient with abnormal uterine bleeding consist of the following:

- Estrogen (premarin)
- Combined oral contraceptives
- NSAIDs
- Antifibrinolytics (tranexamic acid)
- Progesterones
- Androgens
- GnRH-a

The ED treatment of nonpregnancy-related uterine bleeding depends largely on the severity of bleeding, the patient's age, and the potential causes of the bleeding. Patients' access to follow-up care and desire for fertility also affect management choices. Many algorithms require estimation of whether the bleeding has an anovulatory cause or is ovulatory bleeding associated with the menstrual cycle.

Estrogen and combination oral contraceptives

For patients presenting with acute severe bleeding, usually described as menorrhagia (often associated with ovulatory bleeding), causing anemia or hemodynamic instability, recent guidelines suggest the use of high doses of estrogen to get bleeding under control, followed by an oral combination contraceptive taper.[42] Therapeutic options are:

- Premarin (conjugated estrogen)
  - 2.5 mg by mouth every 6 hours, or 25 mg intravenously every 6 hours
- Oral combination pill
  - 30 mg ethinyl estradiol/0.3 mg norgestrel orally 4 times daily until cessation

- ○ 50 mg ethinyl estradiol/0.5 mg norgestrel orally 4 times daily until cessation
- ○ Norethindrone acetate
- ○ Medroxyprogesterone

In the patient with severe bleeding who requires inpatient stabilization and intravenous estrogen, some recommend starting the combination pill simultaneously with premarin. In patients who have milder bleeding and who can be managed as an outpatient, the combination can be started after 48 hours or after bleeding has ceased.

NSAIDs
Nonsteroidal anti-inflammatory medications work by inhibiting cyclooxygenase, which converts arachidonic acids to prostaglandin. When administration of these drugs is initiated during the first 3 days of menses, they decrease overall prostaglandin production and therefore promote vasoconstriction in the uterus, decreasing blood loss.[43] Thus they may be useful for chronic heavy periods or menorrhagia, but their role in acute severe bleeding is less known. One review commented that NSAIDs were superior to placebo at reducing blood loss and were highly significantly more effective at providing "relief from heavy bleeding."[44]

Antifibrinolytics
Tranexamic acid Tranexamic acid is a lysine derivative that prevents fibrin degradation. In 2009, the US Food and Drug Administration approved it for use in patients with menorrhagia. It is administered in a 1.3 g dose three times a day for the first 3–5 days of menses. Tranexamic acid (Lysteda) has been used to treat other bleeding disorders and is believed to be appropriate for women with heavy ovulatory bleeding because they have increased local levels of fibrinolytic activity in the uterus compared with normal patients.[43] Antifibrinolytics decrease bleeding in women with chronic menorrhagia by up to 59%, and have been shown to be superior to NSAIDs and cyclic progestins.[45] Although there has been previous concern that this medication could lead to thromboembolic events such as deep venous thrombosis or pulmonary embolism,[46] a more recent review of the literature does not support an increased risk.[47] However, because there has been inconsistency in the literature, caution should be taken in patients with known thromboembolic history.

Danazol
Androgens such as danazol work by inhibiting steroidogenesis in the ovaries. These agents have several side effects and are limited to 6 months of use. Side effects include weight gain, acne, irritability, headaches, hirsutism, and clitoromegaly. Patients may also experience a decrease in breast size, lipid changes, liver disease, muscle cramps, breakthrough bleeding, and gastrointestinal side effects. A recent Cochrane database review revealed that danazol is more effective than placebo, progestins, NSAIDs, and oral contraceptive pills at reducing blood loss and is more effective than NSAIDs and progesterone-releasing intrauterine devices for shortening the duration of menses, but may have a higher side-effect profile.[48]

Gonadotropin-releasing hormone agonists
GnRH-a are GnRH analogues that work at GnRH receptor sites to create a hypogonadal or hypoestrogen state, resulting in amenorrhea in 3 to 4 weeks. As previously stated, they can be used for the treatment of fibroid-induced menorrhagia, but can be used for only a limited time and are costly. These agents put patients at risk for osteoporosis and cause symptoms similar to menopause, and therefore are often poorly tolerated.

Progesterone

Progestins downregulate estrogen receptors, blunting the effect of estradiol on the endometrium and decreasing endometrial proliferation. Progestins have been used in several delivery methods, including injectables, cyclical oral pill regimens, and intrauterine delivery devices using levonorgestrol, commonly referred to by its brand name Mirena, to control heavy or irregular bleeding. Although the estrogen in combination pills is contraindicated in some women, there are very few contraindications to progesterone treatment.

Cyclical progesterone therapies used on days 14 to 21 have been used to control anovulatory bleeding but have no effect on ovulatory bleeding, and may actually increase blood loss associated with ovulatory bleeding.[43] Examples of cyclical progesterone regimens are:

- Medroxyprogesterone acetate: 5 to 10 mg/d for 10 to 14 days, then repeated for 10 days each month
- Vaginal progesterone gel: intravaginal application every other day between days 17 and 27 of the menstrual cycles has been shown to be as effective as oral progesterone therapy[49]

High-dose continuous progesterone can be used to control or stop bleeding altogether, and is therefore useful in patients with heavy ovulatory bleeding or coagulopathies. Norethisterone (5 mg 3 times daily) and medroxyprogesterone acetate can be given as a 21-day oral course to reduce blood loss substantially and have been shown to reduce blood loss in 87% of patients, but have very poor adherence, making it less superior to the levonorgestrol intrauterine delivery system.[50] Depot medroxyprogesterone acetate (DMPA) is a long-acting subcutaneous injection that is generally more effective, better tolerated, and longer acting than high-dose oral progestins.

Intrauterine progesterone therapy

The levonorgestrol intrauterine delivery device (LNG IUD) (Mirena; Bayer, Montville, NJ) is a T-shaped device that reduces blood loss associated with anovulatory bleeding by 74% to 97%. Many women obtain amenorrhea within 12 months of use. It remains effective in place up to 5 years, and is more effective than norethisterone when used over 21 days of the monthly cycle for reduction of blood loss.[51] Users of the LNG IUD might experience periods of heavier bleeding and spotting during the first 4 months. Compared with hysterectomy and surgical management of abnormal uterine bleeding, the LNG IUD was found to have comparable rates of blood-loss reduction and to provide an overall improved quality of life.[52]

Surgical Treatment

Surgical treatment of abnormal bleeding and menorrhagia is usually reserved for patients in whom medical management and conservative measures are not successful. Dilation and curettage is no longer considered a treatment option because of the high need for recurrent procedures and poor long-term effects. Endometrial ablation can be performed on an outpatient basis under general anesthesia, but the risk to fertility is unknown, so it should not be used in patients wishing to preserve fertility. Hysterectomy achieves the greatest reduction in bleeding, but is definitive. The risk of surgery has to be weighed against the need for it. Surgery should be the treatment of choice for a patient with bleeding associated with endometrial cancer.

SUMMARY

The ED evaluation of patients with acute or chronic vaginal bleeding requires knowledge on the part of the emergency physician regarding the broad differential of underlying causes, options for treatment, and need for gynecologic follow-up. Pregnancy, underlying infection, and structural abnormalities such as fibroids, polyps, and endometriosis should all be considered and evaluated with ultrasound imaging. The severity of bleeding and discomfort will guide the need for appropriate resuscitation, transfusion, and need for outpatient care versus inpatient evaluation. Several first-line medical therapies are used for abnormal bleeding. Knowledge regarding the type of abnormality that is present and the cause of bleeding (anovulatory, ovulatory, or structural) is also necessary for appropriate treatment decisions.

REFERENCES

1. Payson M, Leppert P, Segars J. Epidemiology of myomas. Obstet Gynecol Clin North Am 2006;33:1–11.
2. Parker W. Etiology, symptomatology, and diagnosis of uterine myomas. Fertil Steril 2007;87:725–36.
3. Fischer C, Juhasc-Boess I. Estrogen receptor beta gene polymorphisms and susceptibility to uterine fibroids. Gynecol Endocrinol 2010;26(1):4–9.
4. Yin W, Gore AC. Neuroendocrine control of reproductive aging: roles of GnRH neurons. Reproduction 2006;131:403–14.
5. Munro MG, Critchley HO, Broder MS, et al. The FIGO classification system (PALM-COEIN) for causes of abnormal uterine bleeding in nongravid women in the reproductive years, including guidelines for clinical investigation. Int J Gynaecol Obstet 2011;113:3–13.
6. Munro M. Uterine leiomyomas, current concepts: pathogenesis, impact on reproductive health, and medical, procedural, and surgical management. Obstet Gynecol Clin North Am 2011;38:703–31.
7. Evans P, Brunsell S. Uterine fibroid tumors: diagnosis and treatment. Am Fam Physician 2007;75(10):1503–8.
8. Roche O, Chavan N, Aquilina J, et al. Radiological appearances of gynaecological emergencies. Insights Imaging 2012;3(3):265–7.
9. Hartmann K, Birnbaum H, Ben-Hamadi R, et al. Annual costs associated with diagnosis of uterine leiomyomata. Obstet Gynecol 2006;108:930–7.
10. Gupta S, Manyonda IT. Acute complications of fibroids. Best Pract Res Clin Obstet Gynaecol 2009;23(5):609–17.
11. Bukulmez O, Doody KJ. Clinical features of myomas. Obstet Gynecol Clin North Am 2006;33(1):69–84.
12. Bulun SE. Mechanisms of disease: endometriosis. N Engl J Med 2009;360(3):268–79.
13. Gao X, Outley J, Botteman M, et al. Economic burden of endometriosis. Fertil Steril 2006;86(6):1561–72.
14. Ozkan S, Murk W, Arici A. Endometriosis and Infertility: epidemiology and evidence-based treatments. Ann N Y Acad Sci 2008;1127:92–100.
15. Fourquet J, Gao X, Zavala D, et al. Patients' report on how endometriosis affects health, work, and daily life. Fertil Steril 2010;93(7):2424–8.
16. Stewart WF, Ricci JA, Chee E, et al. Lost productive time and cost due to common pain conditions in the US workforce. JAMA 2003;290:2443–54.
17. Sampson J. The development of the implantation theory for the origin of peritoneal endometriosis. Am J Obstet Gynecol 1940;40:549–57.

18. Sanfilippo JS, Wakim NG, Schikler KN, et al. Endometriosis in association with uterine anomaly. Am J Obstet Gynecol 1986;154(1):39–43.
19. Wittich A. Endometriosis in an episiotomy scar: review of the literature and report of case. J Am Osteopath Assoc 1982;82:22–3.
20. Boyle K, Torrealday S. Benign gynecological conditional. Surg Clin North Am 2008;88:245–64.
21. Karpel J, Appel D, Avraham M. Pulmonary endometriosis. Lung 1985;163(1): 151–9.
22. Burns W, Shencken R. Pathophysiology of endometriosis-associated infertility. Clin Obstet Gynecol 1999;42:586–610.
23. Haney AF. Endometriosis associated infertility. Bailliere's Clin Obstet Gynaecol 1993;7(4):791–812.
24. Beamish R. Postpartum cecal perforation due to endometriosis. JRSM Short Rep 2010;1(7):61.
25. Chapron C, Fauconnier A, Dubuisson JB, et al. Deep infiltrating endometriosis: relation between severity of dysmenorrhea and extent of disease. Hum Reprod 2003;18(4):760–6.
26. Lucidi RS, Witz C. Endometriosis. In: Evans M, editor. Reproductive endocrine and infertility. The requisites in obstetrics and gynecology. Philadelphia: Mosby, Inc; 2007. p. 213–27.
27. Cicchiello L, Hamper UM, Scoutt LM. Ultrasound evaluation of gynecologic causes of pelvic pain. Obstet Gynecol Clin North Am 2011;38:85–114.
28. Buy JN, Ghossain MA, Mark AS, et al. Focal hyperdense areas in endometriomas: a characteristic finding on CT. AJR Am J Roentgenol 1992;159(4):769–71.
29. Stratton P, Winkel C, Premkumar A, et al. Diagnostic accuracy of laparoscopy, magnetic resonance imaging, and histopathologic examination for the detection of endometriosis. Fertil Steril 2003;79(5):1078–85.
30. Moghissi K. Medical treatment of endometriosis. Clin Obstet Gynecol 1999;42: 620–32.
31. Daraï E, Marpeau O, Thomassin I, et al. Fertility after laparoscopic colorectal resection for endometriosis: preliminary results. Fertil Steril 2005;84(4):945–50.
32. Hadfield R, Mardon H, Barlow D, et al. Delay in the diagnosis of endometriosis: a survey of women from the USA and the UK. Hum Reprod 1996;11(4):878–80.
33. Fraser IS, Critchley HOD, Munro MG, et al. Can we achieve international agreement on terminologies and definitions used to describe abnormalities of menstrual bleeding? Hum Reprod 2007;22(3):635–43.
34. Livingstone M, Fraser IS. Mechanism of abnormal uterine bleeding. Hum Reprod Update 2002;8(1):60–7.
35. Warner PE, Critchley HO, Lumsden MA, et al. Menorrhagia I: Measured blood loss, clinical features, and outcome in women with heavy periods: a survey with follow-up data. Am J Obstet Gynecol 2004 May;190(5):1216–23.
36. Sweet MG, Schmidt-Dalton TA, Weiss PM, et al. Evaluation and management of abnormal uterine bleeding in premenopausal women. Am Fam Physician 2012; 85(1):35–43.
37. Madhusoodanan S, Parida S, Jimenez C. Hyperprolactinemia associated with psychotropics—a review. Hum Psychoparmacol Clin Exp 2010;25:281–97.
38. Savaris RF, Braun RD. Menorrhagia and hemoglobin levels. Int J Gynaecol Obstet 2007;97(3):199–200.
39. de Vries CJ, Wieringa-de Waard M, Vervoort CL, et al. Abnormal vaginal bleeding in women of reproductive age: a descriptive study of initial management in general practice. BMC Womens Health 2008;8:7.

40. Dueholm M, Lundorf E, Olesen F. Imaging techniques for evaluation of the uterine cavity and endometrium in premenopausal patients before minimally invasive surgery. Obstet Gynecol Surv 2002;57(6):389–403.

41. Telner D, Jakubovicz D. Approach to diagnosis and management of abnormal uterine bleeding. Can Fam Physician 2007;53(1):58–64.

42. Ely JW, Kennedy CM, Clark EC, et al. Abnormal uterine bleeding: a management algorithm. J Am Board Fam Med 2006;19:590–602.

43. Nelson AL, Teal SB. Medical therapies for chronic menorrhagia. Obstet Gynecol Surv 2007;62(4):272–81.

44. Lethaby A, Augood C, Duckitt K. Nonsteroidal anti-inflammatory drugs for heavy menstrual bleeding. Cochrane Database Syst Rev 2007;(4):CD000400.

45. Wellington K, Wagstaff AJ. Tranexamic acid: a review of its use in the management of menorrhagia. Drugs 2003;63(13):1417–33.

46. Sundström A, Seaman H, Kieler H, et al. The risk of venous thromboembolism associated with the use of tranexamic acid and other drugs used to treat menorrhagia: a case-control study using the General Practice Research Database. BJOG 2009;116(1):91–7.

47. Naoulou B, Tsai M. Efficacy of tranexamic acid in the treatment of idiopathic and non-functional heavy menstrual bleeding: a systematic review. Acta Obstet Gynecol Scand 2012;91(5):529–37.

48. Beaumont H, Augood C, Duckitt K, et al. Danazol for heavy menstrual bleeding. Cochrane Database Syst Rev 2007;(3):CD001017.

49. Karakus S, Kiran G, Ciralik H. Efficacy of micronised vaginal progesterone versus oral dydrogestrone in the treatment of irregular dysfunctional uterine bleeding: a pilot randomised controlled trial. Aust N Z J Obstet Gynaecol 2009;49:685–8.

50. Irvine GA, Campbell-Brown MB, Lumsden MA, et al. Randomised comparative trial of the levonorgestrol intrauterine system and norethisterone for treatment of idiopathic menorrhagia. BJOG 1998;105:592–8.

51. Lethaby A, Cooke I, Rees MC. Progesterone or progestin-releasing intrauterine systems for heavy menstrual bleeding. Cochrane Database Syst Rev 2005;(4). CD002126.

52. Marjoribanks J, Lethaby A, Farquhar C. Surgery versus medical therapy for heavy menstrual bleeding. Cochrane Database Syst Rev 2006;(2):CD003855.

53. Working Party for Guidelines for the Management of Heavy Menstrual Bleeding. An evidence-based guideline for the management of heavy menstrual bleeding. N Z Med J 1999;112:174–7.

54. Lethaby A, Vollenhoven B, Sowter M. Pre-operative GnRH analogue therapy before hysterectomy or myomectomy for uterine fibroids. Cochrane Database Syst Rev 2001;(2):CD000547.

55. Eisinger SH, Bonfiglio T, Fiscella K, et al. Twelve-month safety and efficacy of low-dose mifepristone for uterine myomas. J Minim Invasive Gynecol 2005;12: 227–33.

56. Gupta JK, Sinha AS, Lumsden MA, et al. Uterine artery embolization for symptomatic uterine fibroids. Cochrane Database Syst Rev 2006;(1):CD005073.

57. McPherson K, Metcalfe M, Herbert A, et al. Severe complications of hysterectomy: the VALUE study. BJOG 2004;111:688–94.

Geriatric Gynecology

Karen E. Perkins, MD*, Megan C. King, DO

KEYWORDS

- Postmenopausal vaginal bleeding • Hormone replacement therapy
- Pelvic organ prolapse

KEY POINTS

- Vaginal bleeding in postmenopausal women is the most common presenting symptom of endometrial cancer. Evaluation with transvaginal ultrasound or endometrial biopsy is necessary but can be accomplished on an outpatient basis in stable, reliable patients. If an endometrial stripe of 4 mm or less is observed with ultrasound imaging performed in an emergency department, patients do not need further evaluation of the endometrium.
- Menopause is a physiologic process marked by the cessation of ovarian function and menstrual periods. Hormone replacement therapy (HRT), especially when initiated close to the start of menopause and continued at the lowest possible dose for the shortest duration possible, has less risk than believed previously.
- Pelvic organ prolapse (POP) affects millions of women in the United States and contributes to poor body image and difficulty with urinary, gastrointestinal, and sexual function. Treatment options include Kegel exercises, pessaries, and surgery.

VAGINAL BLEEDING IN THE POSTMENOPAUSAL PATIENT

Vaginal bleeding in premenopausal women is a common patient presentation in emergency departments. When assessing postmenopausal women, an emergency physician's typical patterns of thought regarding gynecologic conditions must be expanded. Postmenopausal bleeding is most commonly defined as vaginal bleeding after a period of no menses for at least 1 year.[1] The physiology of normal menses is contingent on ovulatory cycles, which are marked by endometrial proliferation and secretion and, then, in the absence of pregnancy, a predictable menstrual period after estrogen and progesterone withdrawal.[2] The transition to menopause is often marked by sporadic anovulatory cycles, during which unopposed estrogen stimulates the endometrium and the absence of progesterone results in unpredictable endometrial sloughing and vaginal bleeding. Any bleeding after 1 or more years of no bleeding is

Dr Perkins is now with the Family Medicine Residency, Carilion Clinic, 1314 Peters Creek Road Northwest, Roanoke, VA 24017.
No funding sources or conflicts of interest to disclose.
Family Medicine Department, Medstar Franklin Square Medical Center, 9100 Franklin Square Drive, Baltimore, MD 21237, USA
* Corresponding author. Family Medicine Residency, Carilion Clinic, 1314 Peters Creek Road Northwest, Roanoke, VA 24017.
E-mail address: kperkins@carilionclinic.org

considered abnormal, so further evaluation is required.[1] The more common malignant and benign causes of vaginal bleeding in postmenopausal patients and the evaluation of these patients are reviewed in this article.

Malignant Causes of Vaginal Bleeding

Endometrial cancer

Endometrial cancer is the most common gynecologic malignancy, with a lifetime incidence of 2.6% among women in the United States.[3] Common risk factors include older age, white race, obesity, early menarche, late menopause, nulliparity, infertility, polycystic ovarian syndrome, diabetes, hypertension, hypothyroidism, estrogen therapy without progesterone, tamoxifen use, and hereditary nonpolyposis colorectal cancer (HNPCC). Cigarette smoking and extensive oral contraceptive therapy are protective.[3]

Ninety percent of cases of endometrial cancer are diagnosed in postmenopausal women with vaginal discharge or bleeding. Therefore, this diagnosis should always be considered in this scenario in emergency departments. Not all postmenopausal bleeding indicates cancer, but the likelihood of cancer increases with age.[4]

Endometrial cancer is classified as type I or type II based on histology. Type I (endometriod) is most common, associated with estrogen excess, and carries a better prognosis than type II.[5] Type II endometrial cancer is responsible for approximately 10% of endometrial cancers and includes serous cancer, clear cell carcinoma, and carcinosarcoma.[3]

The precursor lesion of type I endometrial cancer, endometrial hyperplasia, can also cause vaginal bleeding and is graded as follows[3,5]:

- Simple hyperplasia—1% risk of future cancer
- Complex hyperplasia—3% risk of future cancer
- Simple hyperplasia with cellular atypia—8% risk of future cancer
- Complex hyperplasia with atypia—29% risk of future cancer

Therapy for most women with endometrial cancer includes hysterectomy, bilateral salpingo-oophorectomy, retroperitoneal lymph node assessment, and pelvic washings.[3,5] Radiation therapy is controversial for patients with stage I disease, because it does not improve the survival rate, but it is advocated for women with metastatic disease, in combination with chemotherapy.[3] Five-year survival rates for endometrial cancer vary from 91% for cancer limited to the endometrium to 20% for distant metastatic disease.[5] Acceptable therapy for patients with hyperplasia without atypia is progesterone therapy. This treatment can also be offered to women who have atypical hyperplasia or grade 1 endometrial cancer and who desire future fertility, as long as close follow-up (evaluation every 3 months) is ensured.[3]

Ovarian cancer

Ovarian cancer has a lifetime incidence of 1.4% for women in the United States and is the leading cause of gynecologic cancer deaths.[6] Risk factors for ovarian cancer include family history, hereditary breast and ovarian cancer syndrome (BRCA gene mutation), HNPCC, older age (although it can be diagnosed in women of any age), endometriosis, early menarche, late menopause, older age at childbirth, low parity, and a high-fat diet. Multiparity, breastfeeding for greater than or equal to 18 months, oral contraceptive use, and early menopause are protective.[6,7]

The presentation can include vaginal bleeding, but, more commonly, a woman presents with nonspecific symptoms, such as abdominal and pelvic pain, bloating, fullness, dysuria, and early satiety.[6] Most ovarian cancers are epithelial cell in origin and affect older women, whereas the less common stromal cell tumors (5% of cancers) and germ cell tumors (5% of cancers) often affect children and premenopausal women.[7] Prognosis depends on both histology and stage, and standard treatment involves total abdominal hysterectomy, bilateral salpingo-oophorectomy, para-aortic and pelvic lymph node removal, and omentectomy followed by chemotherapy.[7] Survival at 5 years ranges from less than 10% with distant metastatic disease to 99% for cancer limited to one ovary with low malignant potential.[7]

Cervical cancer

Cervical cancer is the third most common gynecologic cancer in the United States. Risk factors include human papillomavirus exposure, early coitarche, smoking, sexually transmitted diseases, immunosuppression, and multiple sexual partners.[8]

The presentation can include postcoital bleeding and vaginal discharge or spotting and the diagnosis can be made via colposcopy and cervical biopsy. Most commonly found at biopsy is squamous cell carcinoma (80%), followed by adenocarcinoma (15%).[8] Unlike endometrial and ovarian cancer, cervical cancer is staged clinically, not surgically. Treatment depends on the stage but often combines surgical therapy with radiation and cisplatin-based chemotherapy. The presence or absence of lymph node metastasis is the most important predictor of survival in early stage cancers; thus, simple hysterectomy alone is appropriate for the earliest microinvasive carcinomas (stage 1a1 [ie, only microscopically visible, 3 mm or less in stromal depth, and 7 mm or less in extension]).[8]

Vaginal cancer

Vaginal cancers are most often metastatic cancers from primary sources, such as the cervix, endometrium, and ovaries. Primary vaginal cancer occurs rarely, accounting for 1% to 2% of gynecologic malignancies, and is associated with risk factors of older age, persistent human papillomavirus infection, vaginal trauma (such as childbirth or hysterectomy), multiple sexual partners, cervical and other gynecologic malignancies, late menarche, early menopause, and smoking.[9]

The presentation is most commonly painless bleeding, with more advanced disease resulting in pelvic pain and possible fistulae.[9] Staging is largely clinical, except for the most advanced disease, and therapy can be either primarily surgical or radiation based and contingent on disease stage, patient age and comorbidities, and the cancer's proximity to other pelvic organs.[9]

Vulvar cancer

Vulvar cancer most typically presents with vulvar pruritus and pain, not vaginal bleeding, and thus is not addressed further.[10]

Benign Causes of Vaginal Bleeding

The statement, "all post-menopausal vaginal bleeding is cancer until proved otherwise," reminds clinicians that a high index of suspicion for cancer is necessary. Most instances of postmenopausal bleeding, however, have benign causes and include but are not limited to the following[2,11–13]:

- Atrophic endometrium
- Cervicitis
- Cervical polyps
- Endometrial polyps
- HRT
- Endometriosis (perimenopausal women)
- Leiomyomas (perimenopausal women)

- Anovulation or oligo-ovulation (perimenopausal women)
- Vaginal atrophy and friability

Evaluation

Patient history

The history should include a risk factor assessment for each type of cancer; for example, an obese, diabetic, nulliparous woman with postmenopausal bleeding has multiple red flags for endometrial cancer. Nonspecific persistent complaints of abdominal pain, bloating, early satiety, and gastrointestinal disturbances merit evaluation for ovarian cancer. Special consideration should be paid to family history, because patients may be at increased risk for BRCA gene mutations or HNPCC syndrome. Perimenopausal women in particular can present a confusing picture, because occasional anovulatory cycles and irregular bleeding can occur for several years before menopause.[14] A patient's social history needs to be addressed as well; a new sexual partner and postcoital bleeding may signify cervicitis from a sexually transmitted disease.

Physical examination

As with any emergency department patient, it is essential to first evaluate the ABCs (airway, breathing and circulation). Special attention should be directed toward hypotension and tachycardia. The general physical examination might reveal indications of advanced cancer, such as unexplained weight loss, decreased breath sounds from a malignant pleural effusion, ascites, or adenopathy.

The gynecologic examination should include a speculum examination to evaluate the cervix for grossly visible lesions and to inspect the vaginal walls for growths suggestive of vaginal cancer (often located in the upper third of the vagina at the posterior wall).[9] The urethra should also be examined to confirm that the bleeding is gynecologic in origin. A bimanual examination performed after patients have voided followed by a rectovaginal examination may improve detection of ovarian or uterine masses. Suggestive findings include fixed masses, ovaries that are palpable 3 to 5 years after menopause, bilateral masses, and nodularity in the cul-de-sac.[15] Unfortunately, the accuracy of the pelvic examination in detecting a mass is limited, particularly in obese women.[16]

Laboratory testing

Laboratory testing should include a complete blood count, a comprehensive metabolic panel, and pregnancy testing in perimenopausal or recently menopausal women.[5,7] Consideration should be given to testing for sexually transmitted diseases in patients at risk for them or with cervicitis. On follow-up from an emergency department visit, patients should be evaluated with a Papanicolaou smear, if deemed appropriate, by a primary care provider. When ovarian cancer is considered a potential cause of vaginal bleeding, a cancer antigen (CA) 125 level should be drawn. The test is most useful in postmenopausal women, because levels can be elevated with common premenopausal conditions, such as uterine leiomyomata, endometriosis, and pelvic inflammatory disease. Higher levels correlate with more advanced disease, and half of women with early epithelial ovarian cancer have a normal CA 125 level.[16]

Imaging

Transvaginal ultrasound is the imaging modality of choice for pelvic structures. Accurate assessment of the endometrium is best obtained immediately after menses in premenopausal patients, when endometrial sloughing has just occurred. In postmenopausal patients on no hormone therapy, an ultrasound scan can be obtained at any time; however, to best evaluate the endometrium, women receiving sequential (but not continuous) HRT should be evaluated immediately after the bleeding from progesterone withdrawal ceases.[1] Stable, reliable patients can be referred to a primary care provider or gynecologist for this ultrasound assessment if the technology is not available in an emergency department.

Endometrial thickness is best measured in the long-axis transvaginal view of the uterus. In postmenopausal patients with atrophic endometrium, it appears as a thin pencil line.[1,15] Endometrial thickness of 4 mm or less measured anterior to posterior in this view is considered normal and highly predictive that no endometrial cancer is present (negative predictive values, 99%–100%).[17] Thus, endometrial sampling is unnecessary and patients can be reassured that their bleeding is not cancerous.

Ovarian evaluation by transvaginal ultrasound supplemented by transabdominal ultrasound for extending masses is the imaging modality of choice for a suspected ovarian mass. Worrisome features on ultrasound include complex masses with cystic and solid components, septated cysts, thick cyst walls, and free fluid in the pelvis.[7] Simple cysts up to 10 cm in diameter have a low chance of malignancy and thus can be followed without intervention in both premenopausal and postmenopausal women.[16] Contrast-enhanced MRI can be used to further evaluate an ovarian mass, but in postmenopausal patients all masses not classified as simple cysts require surgical evaluation.[16]

Endometrial biopsy

Endometrial sampling by a patient's primary care provider or gynecologist is indicated in postmenopausal women with vaginal bleeding and an endometrial thickness greater than 4 mm on ultrasound. Also, women in whom the endometrial stripe cannot be visualized adequately on ultrasound due to obesity, previous uterine surgery, leiomyomata, or axial uterine orientation require an alternate method of evaluation.[15,17] According to the American College of Obstetricians and Gynecologists, it is acceptable to initiate evaluation of postmenopausal vaginal bleeding with endometrial biopsy without ultrasound.[15]

Endometrial sampling is done by dilation and curettage, vacuum aspirator, or suction piston biopsy (ie, endometrial Pipelle, Cooper Surgical, Inc, Trumball, CT, USA). The shortcomings of this procedure include limited ability to sample the uterine cavity, thus introducing the potential to miss focal lesions, such as polyps, endometrial hyperplasia, and cancer.[1]

Postmenopausal women with thickened endometrium on ultrasound with no vaginal bleeding do not require endometrial sampling. This finding is common in this demographic group (10%–17% of these women).[15,17]

MANAGEMENT OF MENOPAUSAL SYMPTOMS

Menopause is infrequently a focus of emergency physicians' training. Emergency physicians are called, however, to diagnose and treat menopausal women on HRT on a regular basis. Menopause is defined as the cessation of menstrual periods for 1 year and occurs at the average age of 51 years.[18] Preceding menopause is often a perimenopausal transition marked by hormonal fluctuations and irregular menses. Although menopause is a normal physiologic process, not a pathologic process, associated symptoms, such as hot flashes, vaginal dryness, poor sleep, and painful intercourse, are irritating to many women.

The discomfort from hot flashes, characterized by intense flushing and sweating lasting for several minutes and potentially occurring multiple times a day, affects 75% of women.[19] Although the exact cause of hot flashes is not known, it is hypothesized that estrogen withdrawal stimulates the release of norepinephrine and serotonin, which in turn alter the body's thermoregulatory mechanism in the hypothalamus, predisposing a woman to more intense fluctuations of body temperature.[19,20] As most women move away from the years immediately surrounding menopause, estrogen levels stabilize and hot flashes abate.

The roles of HRT, including compounded bioidentical hormones, and alternative nonhormonal and herbal remedies for the treatment of menopausal symptoms are discussed.

Hormone Replacement Therapy

The Women's Health Initiative (WHI) study had perimenopausal and menopausal women flocking to physicians for advice on HRT. Beginning in 1993, this study encompassed randomized controlled trials at 40 clinical sites that assessed combined estrogen and progesterone HRT (EPT) in approximately 16,000 menopausal women between the ages of 50 and 79 (mean age, 63) who had an intact uterus.[21] The hormone used was Prempro, a combination tablet of 0.625 mg of conjugated equine estrogen (CEE) and 2.5 mg of medroxyprogesterone acetate. Primary endpoints of coronary heart disease (CHD), invasive breast cancer, stroke, venous thromboembolism (VTE), endometrial cancer, colorectal cancer, and hip fracture were assessed.[21] The combined estrogen and progesterone arm of the study was terminated prematurely after 5 years of follow-up secondary to a documented increased risk of breast cancer, CHD, stroke, and VTE in the group receiving EPT. The risks of colorectal cancer and hip fracture were decreased in this group.[22]

The estrogen-only arm of the WHI enrolled approximately 11,000 women with a history of hysterectomy, who were randomized to receive either placebo or 0.625 mg of CEE (Premarin).[23] Endpoints were the same as for the EPT arm. This study was also terminated prematurely after revealing an increased risk of stroke and VTE in the CEE group. No increased risk of CHD or breast cancer was noted, and a decrease in hip fractures was again seen.[23]

Endpoints from both arms of the WHI study give physicians pause when considering prescribing HRT for menopausal symptoms. Recent guidelines, however, released by the North American Menopause Society (NAMS) suggest that individual risk may be less than suggested by the WHI study when considering a woman's age and the timing of HRT.[24] Also, limitations to the WHI study include older mean age of 63 and the use of only oral estrogen or EPT.[24]

The NAMS 2012 guidelines address the endpoints studied by the WHI as well as several other quality-of-life indicators. The findings and recommendations are summarized here and in **Table 1**[22,24]:

Table 1	
Summary of the risks of hormone replacement therapy	
Medical Condition	**Risk**
CHD	Decreased in younger women (<59 y) Increased when >10 years since menopause
Breast cancer	Increased when EPT used 3–5 y Neutral with estrogen alone
Stroke	Increased in women above 59 y of age
VTE	Increased during therapy for all women
Endometrial cancer	Increased with estrogen alone if patient has a uterus
Colorectal cancer	Decreased with EPT
Bone fracture	Decreased with estrogen and EPT

- CHD
  - Evidence supports the use of HRT, especially estrogen alone, as appropriate in symptomatic younger women when initiated near the time of menopause; HRT reduces CHD risk in these women.
  - CHD risk increases in women who initiate HRT more than 10 years after menopause.
  - HRT is not indicated for the prevention or treatment of CHD in any woman.
- Breast cancer
  - Breast cancer diagnosis is increased when EPT is used for more than 3 to 5 years but not with the use of estrogen alone.
  - A later start of EPT (more remote from the time of menopause) is associated with a lower but still increased risk of breast cancer.
- Stroke
  - Ischemic stroke risk is increased with either estrogen alone or EPT; however, this risk does not translate to women between the ages of 50 and 59 at the initiation of HRT.
- VTE
  - VTE risk is approximately doubled with either estrogen alone or EPT; however, this risk persists only for the duration of therapy.
- Endometrial cancer
  - Unopposed estrogen (without progesterone) in women with a uterus increases endometrial cancer risk; risk is increased with increasing duration of therapy.
  - EPT is recommended instead of estrogen alone for menopausal symptoms in women with a uterus.
- Colorectal cancer
  - EPT decreases the risk of colorectal cancer.
- Fracture
  - HRT decreases all fracture risk but is not approved for the treatment of osteoporosis.
  - Prevention of osteoporosis is an indicated use for HRT, and HRT is recommended in particular patients with premature menopause for bone loss prevention.

The role of progesterone

The NAMS guidelines recommend that all women with a uterus who are taking systemic estrogen therapy should take progesterone therapy as well to decrease the risk of endometrial cancer.[24] This includes oral and transdermal estrogen use but not local intermittent vaginal estrogen therapy.[24] Women without a uterus do not require progesterone therapy.

Although not recommended as primary therapy by the NAMS, progesterone therapy alone has shown benefit for relief of menopausal symptoms in several studies. Both oral megestrol acetate and oral and intramuscular medroxyprogesterone acetate have been beneficial in the reduction of hot flashes compared with placebo.[19] The side effects of progesterone therapy alone include vaginal bleeding, headache, breast tenderness, nausea, and VTE.

Available formulations for HRT

Current estrogen and EPT options include oral pills; transdermal patches, gels, and creams; vaginal creams, rings, and tablets; and intrauterine delivery systems.[22,24] Systemic HRT should involve reassessment yearly for possible tapering/discontinuation of medication as menopausal symptoms abate.

Special considerations

- Premature menopause
  - Premature menopause is diagnosed when it occurs at or before age 40
  - Risks of HRT are less in these young women who are ≤ age 50.
  - Guidelines support HRT in these women until at least the average age of menopause.[24]
- Breast cancer survivors
  - Current standard of care is to avoid HRT in these patients.[19,24]

Bioidentical hormones

Bioidentical hormones are plant-derived hormones that are created by a compounding pharmacy under a physician's direction. They come in various forms, including oral and injectable agents, are not regulated by the US Food and Drug Administration, and have not been subjected to rigorous testing. In general, compounded bioidentical hormones are not recommended for the treatment of menopausal symptoms.[24,25]

Nonhormonal Therapies

Nonhormonal therapies for menopausal symptoms include antidepressants and gabapentin, herbal remedies, and lifestyle modifications. A potential mechanism of action for selective serotonin reuptake inhibitors and norepinephrine serotonin reuptake inhibitors in the treatment of hot flashes is an alteration in the set point of the hypothalamic thermoregulatory zone.[19]

Benefit has been shown from therapy with venlafaxine (Effexor), desvenlafaxine (Pristiq), paroxetine (Paxil), fluoxetine (Prozac), and citalopram (Celexa).[19,20,22] None of these medications, however, carries an indication for the treatment of menopausal symptoms. In general, their benefits (lessening hot flashes by approximately 1 per day) are more modest than those of HRT (lessening hot flashes by 2 or 3 a day).[20] Typical side effects to these medications include drowsiness, nausea, and headache. In addition, there is some concern that certain antidepressants (paroxetine and fluoxetine) can decrease the active metabolite of tamoxifen, endoxifen, which is used in the treatment and prevention of breast cancer. Thus, in patients receiving tamoxifen, menopausal therapy with venlafaxine or citalopram is preferred.[19]

Gabapentin (Neurontin) carries an indication for the treatment of seizures and neuropathic pain. Evidence supports its use for the treatment of hot flashes at a dose of 900 mg daily, with typical side effects of dizziness, dry mouth, and fatigue.[19,20,22] A few studies also show benefit with the use of pregabalin (Lyrica).

Herbal Remedies

Phytoestrogens are plant-derived molecules with estrogenic activity and include products such as isoflavones, lignins, and coumestans.[26] Phytoestrogens are botanic supplements and thus do not undergo the same standardization and testing as do classic pharmaceuticals. Commonly tried remedies for menopausal symptoms are reviewed.

- Soy is an isoflavone with estrogen and antiestrogen properties, found in high concentrations in Asian diets.
  - Some evidence exists for the reduction of hot flashes with soy supplementation, but reports are conflicting.[19,20,26]
  - Soy is not recommended for women with a contraindication to estrogen.[26]
- Black cohosh, derived from the plant *Cimicifuga racemosa*, has been studied as a remedy for hot flashes since the 1980s.

- More recent trials do not support its effectiveness over placebo.[19]
- Flaxseed contains high concentrations of phytoestrogens and may have some benefit in the treatment of hot flashes.[19]
- St. John's Wort has shown benefit in the treatment of depression.[19]

Bioidentical hormones and herbal remedies may carry the same risks as traditional HRT (eg, increased risk of deep vein thrombosis), so emergency physicians should inquire about their use. Rarely should emergency physicians start a patient on HRT or other medication for menopausal symptoms. Instead, they can assure patients that various hormonal and nonhormonal therapies are available for symptom relief and prompt patients to follow-up with a primary care provider or gynecologist.

PELVIC ORGAN PROLAPSE
Definition and Epidemiology

POP refers to the descent of one or more pelvic structures into the vagina. The type of POP is based on anatomic location:

- Anterior (bladder or urethral involvement)
- Posterior (rectal involvement)
- Apical (uterine cervix involvement)

POP is a common problem, but it is often unrecognized by practitioners because patients do not volunteer information and practitioners do not ask the proper questions. Despite possible underdiagnosis, millions of women in the United States are probably affected by this problem, with a predicted 50% increase in prevalence by 2050.[27]

POP can negatively affect patients' quality of life and subsequently contribute to poor psychosocial functioning, leading to anxiety and depression.[28] Body image studies reveal that POP contributes to

- Loss of feelings of femininity
- Loss of feelings of general attractiveness
- Changes in or avoidance of intimacy practices
- Activity modification

Etiology

POP occurs because of weakening of the pelvic floor musculature, which can happen in response to the following[27,29]:

- Vaginal childbirth: increasing parity increases risk (cesarean section is associated with POP as well)
- Increases in intra-abdominal pressure
  - Obesity
  - Straining with chronic constipation
  - Chronic cough (chronic obstructive pulmonary disease)
- Aging/menopause
- Genetic predisposition
- Connective tissue abnormalities

Pathophysiology

POP occurs with the loss of pelvic floor striated muscle support and of connective attachments of the vaginal wall to striated muscles and structures of the pelvis.[30]

The levator ani consists of striated muscle in 3 regions covered by connective tissue that encompasses the superior and inferior fascia of each muscle:

- Iliococcygeal portion—a flat horizontal shelf from one pelvic sidewall to the other
- Pubococcygeus muscle—extends from each pubic bone to the coccyx; attaches to walls of the pelvic organs that traverse it as well as the perineal body
  - Important for suspending the vaginal wall in the pelvis
- Puborectalis—sling around and behind the rectum

In a nonprolapsed state, the muscles have a resting contractile tone that elevates the pelvic floor and prevents prolapse of the pelvic organs by compressing the vagina, urethra, and rectum toward the pubic bone and narrowing the genital hiatus.[30] A recent small study introduced a novel parameter to evaluate POP, which showed that decreased levator ani subtended volume measured with 3-D MRI reconstruction images positively correlated with advancing POP stages defined by the POP question-naire (POP-Q).[31]

Evaluation

History

A main consideration with POP is that if women are not symptomatic, treatment may not be necessary. Often, a practitioner visualizes some degree of prolapse on a pelvic examination, but the patient is asymptomatic. The key piece of history to gather is if a patient feels a bulge in the vagina. If so, other important information should be gathered relating to secondary symptoms—pressure in the vagina, difficulty voiding or stooling, or reports of having to use fingers in the vagina or on the perineum to assist with voiding or stooling.[29]

Physical examination

When examining a patient who reports prolapse, look for a bulge at the vaginal introitus during the Valsalva maneuver. Sometimes it is necessary to have the patient stand and perform the Valsalva maneuver if she describes a bulge that is not visualized in the supine position. If a bulge is present, proceed to systematic evaluation with a speculum:

- Use both blades to examine the cervix and assess for apical prolapse.
- Use the fixed blade only to look at the anterior and posterior vagina individually.
- With examination of each segment, ask the patient to perform a Valsalva maneuver.

Staging

Two systems are commonly used to stage POP[29]:

- Baden-Walker system
  - Grade 0: normal position for each respective site
  - Grade 1: descent halfway to the hymen
  - Grade 2: descent to the hymen
  - Grade 3: descent halfway past the hymen
  - Grade 4: maximum possible descent for each site
- POP-Q
  - Stage 0: no prolapse—anterior and posterior points are all −3 cm and cervix and posterior fornix is between total vaginal length and −2 cm
  - Stage I: the criteria for stage 0 are not met, and the total distal prolapse is more than 1 cm above the level of the hymen

o Stage II: the most distal prolapse is between 1 cm above and 1 cm below the hymen
o Stage III: the most distal prolapse is more than 1 cm below the hymen but no further than 2 cm less than total vaginal length
o Stage IV: represents complete procidentia or vault eversion; the most distal prolapse protrudes to at least 2 cm within the total vaginal length

Treatment Options

Nonsurgical

The first, and cheapest, nonsurgical option is pelvic floor muscle strengthening with Kegel exercises. They are easy to teach and to perform. A practitioner can determine if a patient is isolating the correct muscles either by digital examination or with perineometry. Biofeedback also can be used to teach patients how to isolate the correct muscles. In addition, Kegel cones can be used as an exercise aid.[32] Several studies have demonstrated positive effects of Kegel exercises, both in anatomic and symptomatic measures, especially in patients with mild to moderate prolapse.[27]

The other most commonly known option for nonsurgical treatment of POP is the pessary. Pessaries were once considered only for poor surgical candidates and pregnant women, but they should be considered a treatment option before surgery. They can be fitted by a gynecologist or primary care provider. When proper pessary and size are selected, patients are satisfied with the comfort and the improvement in symptoms. A pessary fits properly when it sits just inside the vaginal introitus and does not fall out with the Valsalva maneuver, urination, or defecation.[27]

Surgical

Surgery remains an option for women in whom nonsurgical treatment was not successful and as a primary option for some. There are open abdominal and laparoscopic approaches as well as options to remove or preserve the uterus. For apical prolapse, options are abdominal sacral colpopexy or transvaginal suspension with the sacrospinous ligament, the uterosacral ligament, or the iliococcygeus fascia/muscle.[29] To avoid hysterectomy, options include uterosacral or sacrospinous ligament fixation by the vaginal approach or sacral hysteropexy by the abdominal approach.[29]

If prolapse is severe and a patient no longer desires vaginal function for either intercourse or childbearing or if the operative risk is too great, colpoclesis (suturing the vaginal opening shut) remains an option.

When anterior or posterior vaginal prolapse is the primary problem, colporrhaphy is used. In these procedures, surgical mesh can be used to augment the procedure. In recent years, much media attention has been directed to the safety of mesh devices. In a joint committee opinion, issued in December 2011, the American College of Obstetricians and Gynecologists and the American Urogynecologic Society outlined the following points[33]:

- Anterior mesh may improve support of the anterior compartment compared with native structures.
- Insufficient data are available for posterior or apical compartments; therefore, it is important to weight risk/benefit for each patient.
- The most common adverse postoperative events are erosion, exposure, extrusion, pelvic pain, groin pain, and dyspareunia.
- Informed consent must be clearly documented with each patient.

SUMMARY

Vaginal bleeding in postmenopausal women is the most common presenting symptom of endometrial cancer. Thus, although vaginal bleeding is often benign, it always merits diagnostic evaluation. Emergency physicians should stabilize patients and perform a complete blood cell count, pregnancy test, speculum examination to evaluate for cervicitis and urogenital lesions, and bimanual examination. Further evaluation with transvaginal ultrasound or endometrial biopsy is necessary but can be accomplished on an outpatient basis in stable, reliable patients. If an endometrial stripe of 4 mm or less is observed with ultrasound imaging performed in an emergency department, a patient does not need further evaluation of her endometrium.

Adnexal masses in postmenopausal patients can be evaluated initially by ultrasound and CA 125 level; however, all suspected masses confirmed on ultrasound, with the exception of simple cysts, require surgical consultation and evaluation.

Menopause is a physiologic process marked by the cessation of ovarian function and menstrual periods. HRT, especially when initiated close to the start of menopause and continued at the lowest possible dose for the shortest duration possible, has less risk than believed previously.

POP affects millions of women in the United States and contributes to poor body image and difficulty with urinary, gastrointestinal, and sexual function. Treatment options include Kegel exercises, pessaries, and surgery.

REFERENCES

1. Goldstein S. The role of transvaginal ultrasound or endometrial biopsy in the evaluation of the menopausal endometrium. Am J Obstet Gynecol 2009;201:5–11.
2. Stovall D. Management of anovulatory bleeding. ACOG Practice Bulletin No. 14. American College of Obstetricians and Gynecologists; 2000 (reaffirmed 2009).
3. American College of Obstetricians and Gynecologists. Management of endometrial cancer. ACOG Practice Bulletin No. 65. Obstet Gynecol 2005;106(2):413–25 (reaffirmed 2011).
4. Ulrich LS. Endometrial cancer, types, prognosis, female hormones, and antihormones. Climacteric 2011;14:418–25.
5. Buchanan E, Weinstein LC, Hillson C. Endometrial cancer. Am Fam Physician 2009;80:1075–80.
6. Clarke-Pearson D. Screening for ovarian cancer. N Engl J Med 2009;361:170–7.
7. Roett M, Evans P. Ovarian cancer: an overview. Am Fam Physician 2009;80(6):609–16.
8. Greer B, Koh W. Diagnosis and treatment of cervical carcinomas. ACOG Practice Bulletin No. 35. American College of Obstetricians and Gynecologists; 2002 (reaffirmed 2010).
9. Lilic V, Lilic G, Filipovic S, et al. Primary carcinoma of the vagina. J BUON 2010;15:241–7.
10. American College of Obstetricians and Gynecologists. Diagnosis and management of vulvar skin disorders. ACOG Practice Bulletin No. 93. Obstet Gynecol 2008;111:1243–50 (reaffirmed 2010).
11. Gale A, Dey P. Postmenopausal bleeding. Menopause Int 2009;15:160–4.
12. Palep-Singh M, Gupta S. Endometriosis: associations with menopause, hormone replacement therapy, and cancer. Menopause Int 2009;15:169–74.
13. American College of Obstetricians and Gynecologists. Alternatives to hysterectomy in the management of leiomyomas. ACOG Practice Bulletin No. 96. Obstet Gynecol 2008;112:387–400.

14. Sweet M, Schmidt-Dalton T, Weiss P, et al. Evaluation and management of abnormal uterine bleeding in premenopausal women. Am Fam Physician 2012;85(1):35–43.
15. American College of Obstetricians and Gynecologists. The role of transvaginal ultrasonography in the evaluation of postmenopausal bleeding. ACOG Committee Opinion No. 440. Obstet Gynecol 2009;113:462–4 (reaffirmed 2011).
16. American College of Obstetricians and Gynecologists. Management of adnexal masses. ACOG Practice Bulletin No. 83. Obstet Gynecol 2007;110(1):201–14 (reaffirmed 2011).
17. Goldstein S. Modern evaluation of the endometrium. Obstet Gynecol 2010;116: 168–76.
18. Perimenopausal bleeding and bleeding after menopause—frequently asked questions—FAQ 162 gynecologic problems. The American College of Obstetricians and Gynecologists; 2011.
19. Pachman DR, Jones JM, Loprinzi CL. Management of menopause-associated vasomotor symptoms: current treatment options, challenges and future directions. Int J Womens Health 2010;2:123–35.
20. Nelson H, Vesco K, Haney E, et al. Non-hormonal therapies for menopausal hot flashes: systematic review and meta-analysis. JAMA 2006;295(17):2057–69.
21. Rossouw J, Anderson G, Prentice R, et al. Risks and benefits of estrogen plus progestin in healthy postmenopausal women: principle results from the women's health initiative randomized controlled trial. JAMA 2002;288(3):321–33.
22. Hill DA, Hill S. Counseling patients about hormone therapy and alternatives for menopausal symptoms. Am Fam Physician 2010;82(7):801–7.
23. Anderson GL, Limacher M, Assaf AR, et al. Effects of conjugated equine estrogen in postmenopausal women with hysterectomy: the women's health initiative randomized controlled trial. JAMA 2004;291(14):1701–12.
24. Gass ML, Heights M, Manson JE, et al. The 2012 hormone therapy position statement of the North American Menopause Society. Menopause 2012;19:257–71.
25. American College of Obstetricians and Gynecologists. Compounded bioidentical hormones. ACOG Committee Opinion No. 322. Obstet Gynecol 2005;106: 1139–40.
26. American College of Obstetricians and Gynecologists. Use of botanicals for management of menopausal symptoms. ACOG Practice Bulletin No. 28. Obstet Gynecol 2001;97(Suppl 6):1–11 (reaffirmed 2010).
27. Culligan P. Nonsurgical management of pelvic organ prolapse. Obstet Gynecol 2012;119:852–60.
28. Lowder JL, Ghetti C, Nikolajski C, et al. Body image perceptions in women with pelvic organ prolapse: a qualitative study. Am J Obstet Gynecol 2011;204: 441.e1–5.
29. American College of Obstetricians and Gynecologists. Pelvic organ prolapse. ACOG Practice Bulletin No. 85. Obstet Gynecol 2007;110:717–29.
30. Word RA, Pathi S, Schaffer JI. Pathophysiology of pelvic organ prolapse. Obstet Gynecol Clin North Am 2009;36:521–39.
31. Rodrigues AA, Bassaly R, McCullough M, et al. Levator ani subtended volume: a novel parameter to evaluate levator ani muscle laxity in pelvic organ prolapse. Am J Obstet Gynecol 2012;206:244.e1–9.
32. Kuncharapu I, Majeroni B, Johnson D. Pelvic organ prolapse. Am Fam Physician 2010;81:1111–7.
33. American College of Obstetricians and Gynecologists. Vaginal placement of synthetic mesh for pelvic organ prolapse. Committee Opinion No. 513. Obstet Gynecol 2011;118:1459–64.

Index

Note: Page numbers of articles titles are in **boldface** type.

Emerg Med Clin N Am 30 (2012) 1021–1028
http://dx.doi.org/10.1016/S0733-8627(12)00091-0
0733-8627/12/$ – see front matter © 2012 Elsevier Inc. All rights reserved.

emed.theclinics.com

United States Postal Service

Statement of Ownership, Management, and Circulation
(All Periodicals Publications Except Requestor Publications)

1. Publication Title
Emergency Medicine Clinics of North America

2. Publication Number
0 0 0 - 7 1 4

3. Filing Date
9/14/12

4. Issue Frequency
Feb, May, Aug, Nov

5. Number of Issues Published Annually
4

6. Annual Subscription Price
$281.00

7. Complete Mailing Address of Known Office of Publication *(Not printer) (Street, city, county, state, and ZIP+4®)*
Elsevier Inc.
360 Park Avenue South
New York, NY 10010-1710

Contact Person
Stephen R. Bushing

Telephone *(Include area code)*
215-239-3688

8. Complete Mailing Address of Headquarters or General Business Office of Publisher *(Not printer)*
Elsevier Inc., 360 Park Avenue South, New York, NY 10010-1710

9. Full Names and Complete Mailing Addresses of Publisher, Editor, and Managing Editor *(Do not leave blank)*

Publisher *(Name and complete mailing address)*
Kim Murphy, Elsevier, Inc., 1600 John F. Kennedy Blvd. Suite 1800, Philadelphia, PA 19103-2899

Editor *(Name and complete mailing address)*
Patrick Manley, Elsevier, Inc., 1600 John F. Kennedy Blvd. Suite 1800, Philadelphia, PA 19103-2899

Managing Editor *(Name and complete mailing address)*
Barbara Cohen - Kligerman, Elsevier, Inc., 1600 John F. Kennedy Blvd, Suite 1800, Philadelphia, PA 19103-2899

10. Owner *(Do not leave blank. If the publication is owned by a corporation, give the name and address of the corporation immediately followed by the names and addresses of all stockholders owning or holding 1 percent or more of the total amount of stock. If not owned by a corporation, give the names and addresses of the individual owners. If owned by a partnership or other unincorporated firm, give its name and address as well as those of each individual owner. If the publication is published by a nonprofit organization, give its name and address.)*

Full Name	Complete Mailing Address
Wholly owned subsidiary of	1600 John F. Kennedy Blvd, Ste. 1800
Reed/Elsevier, US holdings	Philadelphia, PA 19103-2899

11. Known Bondholders, Mortgagees, and Other Security Holders Owning or Holding 1 Percent or More of Total Amount of Bonds, Mortgages, or Other Securities. If none, check box ☐ None

Full Name	Complete Mailing Address
N/A	

12. Tax Status *(For completion by nonprofit organizations authorized to mail at nonprofit rates) (Check one)*
The purpose, function, and nonprofit status of this organization and the exempt status for federal income tax purposes:
☐ Has Not Changed During Preceding 12 Months
☐ Has Changed During Preceding 12 Months *(Publisher must submit explanation of change with this statement)*

PS Form 3526, September 2007 (Page 1 of 3 (Instructions Page 3)) PSN 7530-01-000-9931 PRIVACY NOTICE: See our Privacy policy in www.usps.com

---

13. Publication Title
Emergency Medicine Clinics of North America

14. Issue Date for Circulation Data Below
May 2012

15. Extent and Nature of Circulation

		Average No. Copies Each Issue During Preceding 12 Months	No. Copies of Single Issue Published Nearest to Filing Date
a. Total Number of Copies *(Net press run)*		1228	972
b. Paid Circulation (By Mail and Outside the Mail)	(1) Mailed Outside-County Paid Subscriptions Stated on PS Form 3541. *(Include paid distribution above nominal rate, advertiser's proof copies, and exchange copies)*	685	579
	(2) Mailed In-County Paid Subscriptions Stated on PS Form 3541 *(Include paid distribution above nominal rate, advertiser's proof copies, and exchange copies)*		
	(3) Paid Distribution Outside the Mails Including Sales Through Dealers and Carriers, Street Vendors, Counter Sales, and Other Paid Distribution Outside USPS®	171	128
	(4) Paid Distribution by Other Classes Mailed Through the USPS (e.g. First-Class Mail®)		
c. Total Paid Distribution *(Sum of 15b (1), (2), (3), and (4))*	▶	856	707
d. Free or Nominal Rate Distribution (By Mail and Outside the Mail)	(1) Free or Nominal Rate Outside-County Copies Included on PS Form 3541	74	78
	(2) Free or Nominal Rate In-County Copies Included on PS Form 3541		
	(3) Free or Nominal Rate Copies Mailed at Other Classes Through the USPS (e.g. First-Class Mail)		
	(4) Free or Nominal Rate Distribution Outside the Mail (Carriers or other means)		
e. Total Free or Nominal Rate Distribution *(Sum of 15d (1), (2), (3) and (4))*	▶	74	78
f. Total Distribution *(Sum of 15c and 15e)*	▶	930	785
g. Copies not Distributed *(See instructions to publishers #4 (page #3))*	▶	298	187
h. Total *(Sum of 15f and g)*	▶	1228	972
i. Percent Paid *(15c divided by 15f times 100)*		92.04%	90.06%

16. Publication of Statement of Ownership
If the publication is a general publication, publication of this statement is required. Will be printed in the November 2012 issue of this publication.
☐ Publication not required

17. Signature and Title of Editor, Publisher, Business Manager, or Owner
Stephen R. Bushing
Stephen R. Bushing – Inventory Distribution Coordinator

Date: September 14, 2012

I certify that all information furnished on this form is true and complete. I understand that anyone who furnishes false or misleading information on this form or who omits material or information requested on the form may be subject to criminal sanctions (including fines and imprisonment) and/or civil sanctions (including civil penalties).

PS Form 3526, September 2007 (Page 2 of 3)

EmergencyMed **Advance**

All the latest emergency medicine news and research you need, all in one pla

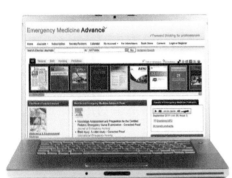

EmergencyMedAdvance.com is a new essential online resource offering valued high-quality content and news for the global community of Emergenc Medicine professionals to save time and stay current—from physicians and nurses to EMTs.

Stay current
• Emergency Medicine news

Save time
• Access relevant articles in press from 16 participating journals

And more...
• Journals' profiles
• Personalized search results
• Emergency Medicine bookstore

• Upcoming meetings and events

• Search across 500+ health sciences journals
• Learn how to submit a manuscript

• Sign up for free e-Alerts
• Emergency Medicine jobs

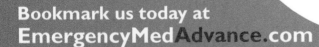